NEW DEVELOPMENTS IN MEDICAL RESEARCH

PULMONARY ARTERIAL HYPERTENSION AND NIFEDIPINE

PATHOGENESIS AND MANAGEMENT

NEW DEVELOPMENTS IN MEDICAL RESEARCH

Additional books in this series can be found on Nova's website under the Series tab.

Additional e-books in this series can be found on Nova's website under the e-books tab.

NEW DEVELOPMENTS IN MEDICAL RESEARCH

PULMONARY ARTERIAL HYPERTENSION AND NIFEDIPINE

PATHOGENESIS AND MANAGEMENT

VICTORIA ESTRADA
EDITOR

NOVA BIOMEDICAL
New York

Library of Congress Cataloging-in-Publication Data

ISBN: 978-1-63482-594-8

Library of Congress Control Number: 2015936751

Published by Nova Science Publishers, Inc. † New York

Contents

Preface

The chapters of this book describe the molecular mechanisms and cellular events regulating vascular remodeling in PAH; the various animal models and drugs currently being used in various laboratories to study mechanisms leading to pulmonary arterial hypertension; and nifedipine, its pharmacology and it's role in the management of pulmonary hypertension and some of the drawbacks concerning its use. The authors also discuss drug delivery systems that can lead to different crystallization forms of the immobilized drug which can lead to better solubility and bioavailability.

Chapter I – Pulmonary arterial hypertension (PAH) is a progressive, fatal syndrome characterized by increased pulmonary vascular resistance that leads to right-ventricular hypertrophy and heart failure, eventually leading to premature death. The prevalence rate of PAH is approximately 25 cases/million/year and the median life expectancy from the time of diagnosis in patients with idiopathic PAH when not treated is 2.8 years. There are no definitive symptoms to identify and confirm PAH until the disease progresses to vascular remodeling and heart failure, and is often associated with poor prognosis. Pulmonary arterial hypertension is characterized by progressive pulmonary vasoconstriction, lumen obliteration of arteries and arterioles, and formation of plexiform lesions. PAH, which leads to pulmonary vascular resistance and right ventricular failure resulting in premature death, is associated with poor prognosis and there is no cure except for treating the symptoms. Vascular remodeling during PAH is the major contributing factor for the advanced stages of the disease. Pathological growth of myofibroblasts from resident fibroblasts and vascular smooth muscle cells, as well as due to endothelial-to-mesenchymal transition (EndMT) in response to transforming growth factor-β (TGFβ) have all been investigated to characterize the underlying reasons for PAH. Aim of this chapter is to describe the molecular mechanisms and cellular events regulating vascular remodeling in PAH.

Chapter II – Pulmonary arterial hypertension (PAH) is a deadly disease with no reliable treatment options available. Uncertainties in the molecular mechanisms and incomplete knowledge on the sequence of events leading to pulmonary arterial hypertension are the major gridlocks in the development of therapeutics for this fatal disease. Research on pulmonary arterial hypertension suffers the lack of proper cellular and animal models. Aim of this chapter is to provide easy to follow protocols supported with clear descriptions of the working principle for each experiment along with a list of all the materials necessary for the successful execution of the experiments. Whereas experimental methods *in vitro* will deal with protocols involved in characterizing the molecular mechanisms leading to fibroblast, endothelial and vascular smooth muscle differentiation into pathological mesenchymal cells. This chapter will also discuss the animal models and drugs currently being used in various laboratories to study mechanisms leading to pulmonary arterial hypertension in rodent and larger animal models.

Chapter III – Nifedipine, a widely prescribed dihydropyridine calcium channel blocker, was originally introduced in 1966 as an anti-anginal drug due to its vasodilatory properties. Subsequently, it was found to have many other properties useful for a variety of indications. Nifedipine – Gastro Intestinal Therapeutic System (GITS) formulation has helped overcoming the main drawback of the drug, which is the sudden drop in blood pressure and reflex tachycardia due to fluctuations in plasma concentrations. Nifedipine has been extensively studied across the world in several robust clinical trials, making available a vast body of information in the literature about its pharmacological properties and therapeutic usage. In addition to its anti-anginal effect, Nifedipine also has an established antihypertensive property. It has been well studied in comparison with a number of drugs belonging to most other major antihypertensive classes, both as solitary and combination therapies. Several trials of Nifedipine studied both general and specific groups of population including the elderly, the diabetics and African Americans. It has been shown to have anti-atherosclerotic, anti-oxidant and vasculo-protectant properties. It reduces the carotid artery intima-media thickness and slows down coronary artery calcification. These are beneficial in the reduction of coronary and cerebrovascular events. Its smooth muscle relaxing function is utilised in the symptomatic treatment of Raynaud's disease. This very function is also utilised in the treatment of ureteric calculi, which could potentially prevent invasive interventions for this condition. Nifedipine is as effective as ACE-inhibitors and angiotensin receptor blockers and could be added as an adjunct to them in protecting renal function in diabetes. It is also comparable to these classes of drugs in reducing left ventricular mass in left ventricular hypertrophy resulting from hypertension. Nifedipine also has utility as a first line tocolytic in prolongation of pregnancy to avoid preterm labor. It is superior to Ritodrine, a beta receptor agonist, in terms of delaying labor, clinically important neonatal outcomes and maternal adverse events.

Chapter IV – Nifedipine has served as one of many advanced therapy options in the treatment of pulmonary hypertension. In comparison to other classes of agents, nifedipine has less adverse effects and can prove to be a preferred option when patients are requiring advanced therapy. In this chapter, the author summarizes the primary and advanced therapeutic options in the management of pulmonary hypertension. Then, the authors focuses on the role of nifedipine with highlights from research studies that have examined the benefits of nifedipine in varying classes of pulmonary hypertension. Lastly, the concept for future studies to examine nifedipine's role in comparison to other advanced therapy agents is introduced and the potential advantages are highlighted.

Chapter V – Calcium channel blockers (CCBs) are widely used for the management of hypertension and angina. Prescription drug sales of CCBs in the United States accounted for US$11.6 billion in 2004, ranking them as the eighth largest drug class in prescription sales. Within this class, Nifedipine, a potent dihydropyridine agent, is widely prescribed accounting for a large share of the annual sales volume. Despite all benefits and versatility presented by such drug (among other counterparts) there are a few drawbacks concerning its use. The main problem with such drug is its low solubility which limits its bioavailability, making it perform less efficiently towards therapeutic use than it can. To circumvent this many research is dedicated to this issue in order to find new polymorphic forms of the drug leading to higher solubility and ultimately to higher bioavailability. On the other hand research is also conducted to develop controlled drug delivery systems bearing in mind that these can lead to better release kinetics, to better patient wellbeing and to better drug resistance and stability to aggressive environmental body conditions (gastric fluids, etc…). Due to confinement effects, such drug delivery systems can also lead to different crystallization forms of the immobilized drug which can lead to better solubility and bioavailability. Recent years have experienced the development of new approaches to prepare such drug delivery systems based on inorganic matrix materials. Taking advantage of the porosity presented by such systems, drugs can be encapsulated becoming then protected and being ready for release. This chapter lights up some recent advances on this niche research topic covering the most relevant advances in the timeframe between 2000 and the present date.

In: Pulmonary Arterial Hypertension … ISBN: 978-1-63482-594-8
Editor: Victoria Estrada

Chapter I

Mechanisms of Vascular Remodeling in Pulmonary Arterial Hypertension

***Harika Sabbineni*[1] *and Payaningal R. Somanath*[1,2,*]**

[1]Clinical and Experimental Therapeutics, College of Pharmacy, University of Georgia and Charlie Norwood VA Medical Center, Augusta, GA, US;
[2]Department of Medicine and Vascular Biology Center, Georgia Regents University, Augusta, GA, US

Abstract

Pulmonary arterial hypertension (PAH) is a progressive, fatal syndrome characterized by increased pulmonary vascular resistance that leads to right-ventricular hypertrophy and heart failure, eventually leading to premature death. The prevalence rate of PAH is approximately 25 cases/million/year and the median life expectancy from the time of diagnosis in patients with idiopathic PAH when not treated is 2.8 years. There are no definitive symptoms to identify and confirm PAH until the disease progresses to vascular remodeling and heart failure, and is often

[*] Corresponding author: Payaningal R. Somanath Ph.D., FAHA, Associate Professor, Clinical and Experimental Therapeutics, College of Pharmacy, University of Georgia, HM1200 – Georgia Regents University, Augusta, GA 30912. Phone: 706-721-4250; Fax: 706-721-3994; E-mail: sshenoy@gru.edu.

associated with poor prognosis. Pulmonary arterial hypertension is characterized by progressive pulmonary vasoconstriction, lumen obliteration of arteries and arterioles, and formation of plexiform lesions. PAH, which leads to pulmonary vascular resistance and right ventricular failure resulting in premature death, is associated with poor prognosis and there is no cure except for treating the symptoms. Vascular remodeling during PAH is the major contributing factor for the advanced stages of the disease. Pathological growth of myofibroblasts from resident fibroblasts and vascular smooth muscle cells, as well as due to endothelial-to-mesenchymal transition (EndMT) in response to transforming growth factor-β (TGFβ) have all been investigated to characterize the underlying reasons for PAH. Aim of this chapter is to describe the molecular mechanisms and cellular events regulating vascular remodeling in PAH.

Introduction

"Pulmonary arterial hypertension (PAH) is a progressive, fatal syndrome characterized by increased pulmonary vascular resistance that leads to right-sided heart failure and, eventually, death" (Rosanio et al., 2014) A mean pulmonary artery pressure (PAP) of >25 mmHg, pulmonary vascular resistance >3 Wood units, pulmonary capillary wedge pressure <15 mmHg, and normal or reduced cardiac output in absence of other causes of pulmonary hypertension is regarded as PAH (Galie et al., 2009) The term pulmonary hypertension (PH) refers to a condition with abnormally high pulmonary vascular pressure. It is important to note that PAH is a sub-category of PH and the two terms are not synonymous.

Pulmonary arterial hypertension results from restricted blood flow through the pulmonary arterial circulation resulting in increased pulmonary vascular resistance ultimately causing right sided heart failure. During the past few decades of extensive research on mechanisms contributing to the development of PAH, multiple pathogenic pathways have been implicated, including those at the molecular and genetic levels in the endothelial cells, vascular smooth muscle cells, and fibroblasts. It has been believed until recently that the imbalance in the vasoconstrictor/vasodilator milieu served as the root cause for the development of PAH and hence the basis for current medical therapies, although increasingly it is recognized that an imbalance of proliferation and apoptosis contributes to PAH.

While previously considered a rare disease, recent evidence suggests that the prevalence of PAH is about 15 per million (Humbert et al., 2004) There is no cure for this fatal disease which affects mainly young to middle aged women and survival rate is estimated at 55-65% 3 years post diagnosis despite recent improvements in PAH therapies.(Stacher et al., 2012) It is associated with poor prognosis, with an approximately 15% mortality within 1 year on modern therapy.(Thenappan, Shah, Rich, & Gomberg-Maitland, 2007) A few predictors of a poor prognosis include: advanced functional class of the disease, poor exercise capacity as measured by 6-minute walk (6MW) test or cardiopulmonary exercise test, high right atrial (RA) pressure, significant right ventricular (RV) dysfunction, evidence of RV failure, low cardiac index, elevated brain natriuretic peptide (BNP), and underlying diagnosis of scleroderma spectrum of diseases.

Classification

Based on the World Health Organization (WHO) classification, PAH constitutes the first class of pulmonary hypertension (PH) and it comprises two different forms (WHO Group 1): a) Idiopathic PAH which is more prevalent in women and was the most commonly reported type of PAH in the French registry and, b) Heritable/Familial PAH which often results from a mutation in the bone morphogenic protein receptor-2 (BMPR2) and is inherited as an autosomal dominant disease. Other genetic mutations contributing to the development of familial PAH include activin receptor-like kinase-1, endoglin, decapentaplegic 9, caveolin-1, or KCNK3. Familial PAH may also be induced by anorexigen, medical conditions associated with PAH including portal hypertension, connective tissue disease, human immunodeficiency virus, schistosomiasis, chronic hemolytic anemia, and congenital heart disease. Besides WHO Group 1 PAH, other forms of pulmonary hypertension include WHO Groups 2 (pulmonary venous hypertension or pulmonary hypertension associated with left heart disease), 3 (pulmonary hypertension associated with lung diseases and/or hypoxemia), 4 (pulmonary hypertension due to chronic thrombotic and/or embolic disease), and 5 (pulmonary hypertension due to miscellaneous or multifactorial causes) (Simonneau et al., 2013)

Symptoms and Diagnosis

The most commonly reported physiological symptoms of PAH are shortness of breath, dyspnea on exertion, and fatigue. Other symptoms may include syncope, chest pain, abdominal distention, and peripheral edema (Barst et al., 2004) PAH may also present psychological symptoms including anxiety, depression, panic attacks, and panic disorders (Looper, Pierre, Dunkley, Sigal, & Langleben, 2009; Lowe et al., 2004)

Over the last decade, the age at diagnosis of PAH has been gradually shifting to older age (Hoeper, Huscher, et al., 2013) while the mean age of diagnosis is 50 years (Badesch et al., 2010). Patients at a great risk for the development of PAH who need to be screened periodically include those with a known mutation in BMPR2, scleroderma spectrum of diseases, and portal hypertension. The most fundamental principles in the diagnostic workup of patients with clinical suspicion of PH/PAH remain unchanged over years. Any patient who presents with otherwise unexplained dyspnea on exertion, syncope, and/or signs of right ventricular dysfunction should be suspected of PAH and screened immediately. By far, the most appropriate study to obtain in patients suspected of having PH based on physical examination, medical history, chest x-ray (CXR), and electrocardiogram (ECG) is an echocardiogram. Transthoracic echocardiography continues to be the most important noninvasive screening tool but right heart catheterization (RHC) remains mandatory to establish the diagnosis. RHC is the gold-standard procedure for the diagnosis and classification of pulmonary hypertension and is recommended for all patients suspected of having PAH before the initiation of any PAH-specific therapy and should include measurement of pulmonary artery pressure, pulmonary wedge pressure, cardiac output, and oxygen saturations in the central veins, cardiac chambers, and pulmonary artery; calculation of pulmonary vascular resistance; and performance of vasodilator testing. (Hoeper, Bogaard, et al., 2013; McLaughlin et al., 2009) Acute vasodilator testing should be performed in all IPAH patients who might be considered potential candidates for long-term calcium-channel blocker therapy. It involves administration of pharmacologic agents to test the presence of pulmonary vasoreactivity and should not be performed on patients with right heart failure or hemodynamic instability.(McGoon et al., 2004) Evaluation for other potential etiologies, such as thromboembolic disease, is appropriate in all patients suspected of having PAH.

In a very recent study, Staniszweska-Slezak et al., demonstrated that FTIR spectroscopy supported by principal component analysis (PCA) has the potential to become a fast and non-destructive method for biochemical characterization of plasma that consequently could have a diagnostic significance in pulmonary arterial hypertension (Staniszewska-Slezak et al., 2015)

Biomarkers

Given our incomplete understanding of the pathogenesis, heterogeneity and complexity of PAH, numerous markers have been investigated for their potential as biomarkers. However, almost none of those markers studied has been identified and validated as clinically relevant to diagnose PAH. Many circulating biomarkers have the potential of informing clinical prognosis, guiding therapeutic decisions, and/or providing other unique information relevant to PH patients. There should be general and inter-lab reproducibility, relevance to the disease process, cost-effectiveness, and validation, preferably with good external validity for a biomarker to be successfully employed in diagnosis and treatment. Brain natriuretic peptide (BNP) or the N-terminal fragment of pro-BNP (NT-proBNP) is the only biomarker recommended by current guidelines for risk stratification where a "normal" BNP is suggested as a treatment goal addressing endpoints for PAH treatment.(Galie et al., 2009). Following are a few markers that have the potential of being employed as biomarkers for PAH if investigated further and proven successful.

Nitric oxide (NO) - NO is an important endogenous vasodilator which acts in part through the activation of soluble guanylate cyclase (sGC) causing vascular smooth muscle cell relaxation. The lungs of patients with PAH showed reduced expression of eNOS which might be an evidence for the concept of deficient NO as a pathogenic factor in PAH. However, few groups have reported a regional distribution of high levels of eNOS enzyme in the plexiform lesions of patients with PAH.

Asymmetric and symmetric dimethylarginines (ADMA and SDMA) - Asymmetric dimethyl arginine (ADMA) and symmetric dimethyl arginine (SDMA) are methylarginines that inhibit NO synthesis. Serum levels of both ADMA and SDMA are known to be elevated in patients with Group I PAH. This may be associated with a decrease in the enzyme dimethylarginine dimethylaminohydrolase (DDAH) that degrades ADMA. ADMA levels were elevated in patients with chronic thromboembolic pulmonary hypertension (CTEPH) and correlated with mixed venous oxygen saturation, right atrial pressure, and cardiac index.

NO and exhaled NO (eNO) in PAH - The biological half-life of NO varies between 0.1 and 5 seconds, hence limiting its use as a potential biomarker. Although few animal studies showed that exhaled NO (eNO) represents NO production from the pulmonary circulation, the credibility of eNO being employed as a measurement of NO is still debatable because some studies have demonstrated local underproduction of NO in exhaled airway gas from patients with PAH while others have demonstrated normal values.

NOx: nitrite and nitrate - Nitrite (NO2-) and nitrate (NO3-) referred to as NO metabolites (NOx) are oxidized products of NO. Measurement of NOx as a surrogate of in vivo NO activity has been of interest. However, the use of these metabolites as biomarkers for PAH is challenging because their levels are significantly affected by dietary factors, and glomerular filtration and plasma NOx levels in PAH patients have been variable. Further investigation is necessary to critically evaluate and characterize the potential role of these biomarkers in assessing severity and response to treatment in PAH.

Red blood cell (RBC) S-nitrosothiols (SNO) - NO reversibly binds to a thiol sulfur of the cysteine residue of the hemoglobin (Hb), forming an S-nitroso-Hb (SNOHb). The S-nitrosothiol (SNO) side group is effectively released and exported from the RBC to mediate intercellular signaling when deoxygenation triggers the conformational switch in hemoglobin from the oxygenated “R” structure to the deoxygenated “T” structure, in which NO/SNO binding is no longer favored. Decreased RBC SNO levels are reported in patients with advanced PAH.

cGMP - cGMP is an intracellular secondary messenger found in platelets, vascular smooth muscle and other cells. Several groups have reported that urinary cGMP levels are higher in PAH patients compared to healthy controls or patients with asthma, and correlated inversely with cardiac index. The elevated cGMP in Group I PAH presumably reflects GC activation by BNP and/or ANP, rather than by bioactive NO and its derivatives, which may be depressed in PAH.

cAMP - cAMP is a second messenger in various cell types that are responsible for the modulation of vascular remodeling in PAH. Intracellular cAMP in human pulmonary arterial smooth muscle cells is elevated by iloprost and treprostinil which are FDA approved prostacyclin analogues.

NT-Pro-BNP and NT-ANP - The first biomarkers identified in PAH patients were natriuretic peptides. BNP, primarily released from the heart is involved in natriuresis and vasodilation via the renin/angiotensin pathway. Atrial natriuretic peptide (ANP) is secreted from cardiac atria in response to increased atrial pressure, as is the N-terminal of ANP (NT-ANP). In a recent study, Wiedemann et al. identified significantly elevated baseline ANP levels in PAH patients compared to healthy controls which correlated with baseline right atrial pressure, pulmonary vascular resistance (PVR), and mixed venous O2 saturation of hemoglobin. (Wiedemann et al., 2001) This was further supported by a decrease in ANP levels in patients with PAH upon treatment with iloprost, which correlated with decreases in mean pulmonary PAP and PVR. BNP is more stable and less sensitive to temperature changes, making it a more practical test than ANP. Further, metabolic clearance of NT-proBNP is slower and hence has an advantage over BNP.

Endothelin-1 (ET-1) and CT-proET-1 - Endothelin-1 (ET-1) is a potent vasoconstrictor that stimulates proliferation of pulmonary artery smooth muscle cells (SMCs). Plasma levels of both ET-1 and its precursor, big ET-1 correlated with pulmonary vascular resistance (PVR), mean pulmonary artery pressure, cardiac output, cardiac index, and six minute walk distance; while levels of ET-1 also correlated with right atrial pressure, indexed PVR, cardiac index and mixed venous oxygen saturation. Given its longer circulating half-life, Big ET-1 might be a more reliable biomarker than ET-1.

Matura et al. showed in a study that circulating inflammatory biomarkers such as interleukin-6(IL-6) and tumor necrosis factor-alpha(TNF-α) were significantly associated with increased bodily pain and other quality of life related symptoms in PAH patients.(Matura et al., 2015)

In addition to the ones discussed above, the biomarkers that need to be further investigated to evaluate their potential of being reliable biomarkers to diagnose PAH include uric acid, bilirubin, creatinine, isoprostanes, C-reactive protein, osteopontin, osteoprotegerin, growth differentiation factor-15, herat type fatty acid binding protein, lowered HDL, troponin, thrombomodulin, factor VIII, soluble CD40 ligand, addrenomedullin, angiopoetin-2, platelet derived growth factor, vascular endothelial growth factor and circulating endothelial cells.(Swaminathan, Dusek, & McMahon, 2015)

Pathogenesis of PAH

The major factors contributing to increased pulmonary vascular resistance in PAH include vasoconstriction, proliferative, and obstructive remodeling of the pulmonary vessel wall, inflammation, resistance to apoptosis, formation of plexiform lesions, and thrombosis *in situ.* (Christman et al., 1992; Farber & Loscalzo, 2004; Giaid & Saleh, 1995; Giaid et al., 1993; Humbert et al., 2004) A common feature to all vascular remodeling processes is that in early stages of the disease, a significant increase in oxidative stress and inflammatory processes are observed, causing irreversible DNA damage and cell death. This leads to 1) endothelial injury and 2) enhanced inflammatory response, which could be the underlying causes of exaggerated vasoconstriction and vascular cell proliferation and contribute to the occlusive pulmonary vascular remodeling that characterizes PAH. (Montani et al., 2013; Wojciak-Stothard et al., 2014)

i) Role of Endothelial Cells and Their Cross Talk with Different Cell Types in Vasculature

Endothelial Response to Injury

Endothelial injury is believed to be the first insult that triggers vascular remodeling in PAH. The endothelial response to injury results in an initial/rapid response followed by a phenotypic response.(Sitbon et al., 2005) The initial response is rapid and involves changes in levels of nitric oxide (NO), endothelin-1 (ET-1), thromboxane, and 5-hydroxytryptamine (5-HT) leading to initial pulmonary artery endothelial cell (PAEC) apoptosis, disruption of the endothelial layer, and exposure of the subendothelium to soluble growth factors and cytokines. This is followed by a phenotypic response in which the apoptotic endothelial cells release mediators that not only promote the survival of surrounding endothelial cells, which undergo disordered proliferation along with aberrant neoangiogenesis but also affect the underlying basement membrane and the PA smooth muscle cells (PASMCs). Endothelial lesions can be seen as an integrative hub triggering multiple pathophysiological pathways which are well recognized signals in cardiovascular diseases, including PAH. (Lannan, Phipps, & White, 2014; Newby, 2006)

Endothelial Dysfunction and Vasoconstriction/Vasodilatation

Endothelial dysfunction leads to sustained vasoconstriction of the pulmonary circulation via loss of homeostasis between vasodilators and vasoconstrictors such as NO, ET-1, thromboxane, and 5-HT there by affecting contraction and relaxation of PASMCs. Because of the complexity of signaling integration by PASMCs, the mechanism by which they respond to these stimuli is not clearly known. The signaling pathways affected by these vasoactive molecules is not restricted to the classical K+ channel/Ca2+ channel axis (Li et al., 2012; Thomas, Ciuclan, Hussey, & Press, 2013) indeed, it was recently shown that chronic hypoxia increases transient receptor potential vanilloid 4, which is overexpressed in PAH, and mobilizes calcium in response to 5-HT resulting in PASMC vasoconstriction. (Xia et al., 2013) In addition to this vasoconstrictive effect NO downregulation causes vasodilatation impairment in distal pulmonary arteries by a still elusive mechanism. The altered NO levels in the PAs affect the PAECs only, since the PAH-PASMCs do not sense NO because of the upregulation of phosphodiesterase 5, leading to degradation of second messenger of NO and hence impairment of vasodilatation. Together, it is evident that gene expression in PASMCs depends on the stimulation of PAEC.

Endothelial Dysfunction and Impaired Angiogenesis

NO downregulation and increased ET-1 in ECs lead to vasoconstriction and selection of a proproliferative and antiapoptotic EC population. Upregulation of ET-1 reduces the expression of peroxisome proliferator-activated receptor (PPAR)-γ, resulting in decreased endothelial NO synthase (eNOS) expression, reduced tube formation, and hence impaired angiogenesis (Guignabert et al., 2009) and (Wolf et al., 2014) Interestingly, Potus et al. (Potus et al., 2014) showed decreased angiogenesis in peripheral muscles of PAH patients driven by decreased microRNA (miR)-126 expression in ECs. It was also shown that activation of c-Jun N-terminal kinase/c-Jun by epoxyeicosatrienoic acid in cultured ECs leads to an increase in proliferation and tube formation, suggesting a potential promotion of angiogenesis in PAH.(Ma et al., 2012) However, the exact role of angiogenesis in PAH remains elusive. It could be hypothesized that early in the disease, the apoptosis of PAECs contributes to a decrease in angiogenesis, and in the later stage PAEC hyperproliferation contributes to an increase in angiogenesis and thus contribute to plexiform lesion (PL) formation.

Endothelial Dysfunction and Plexiform Lesions

Formation of plexiform lesions (PL) is a hallmark characteristic of severe PAH. PLs are complex glomeruloid-like vascular structures originating from the distal PAs whose development depends on the progressiveness and severity of PH. (Abe et al., 2010) Although the cellular composition of PLs is highly debatable, it is widely believed that they are constituted of highly proliferative ECs and myogenic interstitium which are plastic and their phenotype changes according to their environment. PLs express high messenger RNA (mRNA) levels of angiotensin II, hypoxia-inducible factor (HIF) 1-α, matrix metalloproteinase (MMP) 9, vascular endothelial growth factor (VEGF) α and its receptors. Surprisingly, ECs composing PLs exhibit several neoplastic characteristics including high proliferation rate, resistance to apoptosis, modified mitochondrial metabolism (Warburg-like), and increased DNA damage. However, the molecular mechanism underlying PL formation and the series of events that are triggered remain unclear. Recently, translationally controlled tumor protein (TCTP), a well known tumor promoting mediator was shown to be involved in prosurvival and growth signaling of ECs in PAH.(Rubens et al., 2001) Also, it has been proposed that DNA mutations might contribute to the development of the neoplastic phenotype observed in PAH-PAECs that might occur through shear stress, oxidative stress, and increased inflammation, all of which play critical role in the etiology of PAH.

ii) Role of Inflammation and Autoimmunity

Inflammation is critical in pathogenesis of PAH by contributing to vascular remodeling that correlates with vascular thickening. The inflammatory environment is characterized by the presence of increased inflammatory cells, cytokines, and chemokines which exacerbate the inflammatory response.

Inflammatory Cells

Many immune cells are highly upregulated in PAH, such as T and B lymphocytes and macrophages. T cells are essential components of adaptive immunity. Several studies suggest that T cells are not only a part of vascular remodeling but also the initiators ("initial hit"). Cuttica et al. demonstrated in a Rag1tm1Mom mouse model that perivascular inflammation composed mainly of helper T lymphocytes that preceded pulmonary arterial remodeling.(Cuttica et al., 2011) Activated B cells in PAs and PLs contribute to the immune regulation through various mechanisms including antigen presentation, cytokine and autoantibody production. Interestingly, anti-EC antibodies might play a critical role in PAH pathogenesis by inducing the expression of adhesion molecules and apoptosis of ECs. It has been reported that the number of macrophages which produce leukotriene B4 that induces apoptosis of PAEC and proliferation and hypertrophy of PASMC increased in PLs and in perivascular inflammation of IPAH lungs. Satoh et al. showed that upregulation of the receptor basigin (Bsg) in lungs of PAH patients was involved in the increase of macrophages and production of cytokines/chemokines and that high levels of its ligand, cyclophilin A, was associated with poor outcome. Through Bsg extracellular cyclophilin A activates extracellular signal-regulated kinase (ERK) 1/2 in vascular smooth muscle cells, and induces the production of pro-inflammatory cytokines (IL-1β, IL-2, TNF-α, etc), chemokines and platelet-derived growth factor (PDGF).(Satoh et al., 2014) *In vivo*, studies using hypoxia induced PAH model showed that a deficiency in Bsg improved the outcomes. In a chronic hypoxia rat model, Choi et al. demonstrated the anti-inflammatory properties of melatonin which acts via suppression of nuclear factor-κB, a transcription factor that is highly upregulated in PAH and is a key regulator of pro-inflammatory cytokines and macrophage activation. By decreasing the phosphorylation of protein kinase B (also known as Akt, PKB/Akt) and ERK1/2, melatonin inhibited PASMC proliferation and hence attenuated pulmonary vascular remodeling.(Choi et al., 2011)

Cytokines and Chemokines

In PAH, the levels of cytokines (IL-6, IL-1, TNF-α) and chemokines (fractalkine) which have been shown to be key players in PAH pathogenesis by modulating various process contributing to vascular remodeling such as proliferation, differentiation, and migration of pulmonary vascular cells are increased. Increased IL-6 levels induce pericyte migration and vascular remodeling via activation of signal transducer and activator of transcription 3(STAT3) and Krüppel-like factor 5 (KLF). IL-1 also plays an important role in vascular remodeling by regulating osteoprotegerin secretion by PASMCs, which induces cell proliferation and migration. TNF-α inhibits pyruvate dehydrogenase (PDH) and hence regulates the apoptosis-resistant phenotype of PASMC, which contributes to mitochondrial membrane hyperpolarization and nuclear factor of activated T cells (NFAT) activation.(Sutendra et al., 2011) High levels of TNF-α induce IL-6 and phosphodiesterase-1c protein expression in PAs and macrophage infiltration in the lungs of a cold-induced PH animal model, all of which were decreased with TNF-α short hairpin small interfering RNA therapy suggesting a potential role of cytokines and chemokines in the pathogenesis of PAH.(Crosswhite, Chen, & Sun, 2014)

Molecular Mechanisms Contributing to PAH-PASMC and PAEC Proliferation and Resistance to Apoptosis

In order to develop an effective treatment strategy, it is very important to understand the molecular mechanisms that trigger and maintain the PASMC and PAEC proliferation/apoptosis imbalance which greatly contributes to vascular remodeling and hence the development of PAH.

The Src/STAT3 Integrative Hub

In PAH, there is a high turnover of hyperproliferative and apoptosis-resistant PASMC and PAEC populations which contribute to PA remodeling. Several mechanisms have been identified as important players in this proliferation/apoptosis imbalance of which the most described pathway is the transforming growth factor (TGF) β pathway. Mutations in bone morphogenic protein receptor 2 (BMPR2), a member of the TGF-β superfamily are found in 50% of familial PAH cases and disruption of this pathway is most commonly found in other forms of PAH as well.(Austin & Loyd, 2014) Mutations in the BMPR2 gene activate the v-Src sarcoma (Schmidt-Ruppin A-2 [Src]) pathway, leading to subsequent activation of downstream signal transduction pathways including STAT3 which leads to a disruption of the BMPR2 pathway. Additionally, cytokines and growth factors such as PDGF and VEGF also activate STAT3 by binding to tyrosine kinase receptors. From the wealth of literature it is evident that the Src/STAT3 axis is a central integrative hub in PAH which controls multiple pathways implicated in PASMC and PAEC proliferation, migration, and resistance to apoptosis. In addition to affecting BMPR2, Src/STAT3 also regulates several signaling molecules including NFATc2, HIF-1, survivin, provirus integration site for Moloney murine leukemia virus-1 (Pim-1), and matrix metalloproteinases (MMP). It is important because overexpression of Pim-1/NFATc2 upregulates PASMC proliferation by promoting mitochondrial hyperpolarization and antiapoptotic proteins, such as survivin. The extracellular matrix modifiers MMPs, notably MMP-2 and MMP-9 play a significant role in PAH vascular remodeling by promoting PAEC and PASMC proliferation and migration. Src/STAT3 activation also regulates PASMC migration via phosphorylation of focal adhesion kinase (FAK). Therapeutically, inhibition of the Src/STAT3 pathway has been shown to reverse the PAH phenotype in many pre-clinical studies.

Metabolic Switch: The Warburg Effect

Very similar to cancer, PAH-PASMCs and -PAECs are driven by several metabolic changes that promote their proproliferative and antiapoptotic phenotype. One of the major metabolic changes includes the switch from oxidative phosphorylation to glycolysis, also known as Warburg effect which leads to greater glucose uptake by the affected cells. A greater lung glucose uptake in PAH subjects compared with in the control subjects has been reported in a recent study, confirming the Warburg effect in PAH. (Cottrill & Chan, 2013)

Although establishment of the Warburg effect in PAH remains unclear, recent evidence has suggested that endoplasmic reticulum (ER) stress that induces mitochondrial enzyme dysfunction and impairs metabolism might be a contributing factor. Indeed, hypoxia, mutations in BMPR2, and inflammation all of which trigger PAH, increase the expression of neurite outgrowth inhibitor (Nogo) B via the activating transcription factor 6 (ATF6), an ER stress-regulated transcription factor. Nogo-B is a regulator of the ER structure that increases the distance between ER and mitochondria, thus decreasing ER-to-mitochondria phospholipid transfer and intramitochondrial calcium. This results in an increased mitochondrial membrane potential and decreased PDH expression, reactive oxygen species production, and mitochondrial-dependent apoptosis. Activation of transcription factors such as STAT3, HIF-1, or NFAT further sustains this phenotype. Together, warburg effect is advantageous for the development of PAH as it promotes increased expression of proliferative factors and availability of nutrients, decreased mitochondrial-dependent apoptosis, and regulates epigenetic mechanisms.

Epigenetic Mechanisms of PH

Epigenetics, the study of molecular mechanisms implicated in the regulation of gene expression at genome level, without modification of the DNA sequence is a fast growing area of research in many diseases, particularly PAH. The major epigenetic phenomena include microRNAs (miRNAs), DNA methylation, and histone modifications.

Role for miRNAs

MiRNAs are small non-coding RNAs consisting of 20-23 nucleotides targeting a specific pool of mRNAs, resulting in their degradation. Several studies suggest an interesting role for miR-204 in vascular remodeling in PAH, because it regulates the Src/STAT3 axis which is highly implicated in the pathogenesis of PAH.(Bienertova-Vasku, Novak, & Vasku, 2014; Courboulin et al., 2011) Recently, it was demonstrated that the expression of miR-130/301 is upregulated in different PAH models sustaining the PAH-PASMC proproliferative antiapoptotic phenotype and its activation results in downregulation of miR-204. It is interesting because upregulation of miR-130/301 increases the fibroblast growth factor (FGF) expression via PPARγ which is involved in inducing a metabolic switch in PAECs, thus suggesting a role for the miR-130/301/PPARγ axis in the glycolytic switch observed in PAH-ECs.(Bertero et al., 2014)

It has been reported that other miRNAs, such as miR-145, miR-17/92 cluster, are associated with the complexly disrupted BMPR2 signaling in PAH.(Brock et al., 2014) In a recent study, Caruso et al. demonstrated that miR-145 expression is increased in lungs and right ventricles of the mice which were exposed to chronic hypoxia to induce PAH which was in agreement with increase in miR-145 in lungs of IPAH and heritable PAH patients.(Caruso et al., 2012) This was supported by their observation that miR-145 knockout mice are resistant to PAH development under hypoxia. However, miR-145 expression is decreased in PLs, which regulates the phenotypic switch of SMC from the differentiated to the proliferative state via various transcription factors. In PLs, they also reported a decrease in the expression of miR-126, an angio-miR mainly expressed by ECs.(Goerke, Kiefer, Stark, Simunovic, & Finkenzeller, 2014) This is in total agreement with the observations of Potus et al. that there is a decreased miR-126 expression in decompensated right ventricle (RV) and peripheral muscle of PAH patients which results in an upregulation of sprouty-related EVH1 domain enabled/VASP homology 1 domain-containing protein 1 and hence impairment of angiogenesis. The miR-17/92 cluster that is transcriptionally regulated by STAT3 that targets BMPR2 which inturn regulates miR-21 has been implicated in EC angiogenesis, and might thus play an important role in endothelial injury. miR-21 suppresses Rho/Rho kinase activity, leading to decreased angiogenesis and vasodilatation.(Parikh et al., 2012) Additionally, a decrease in the expression of miR-193 is observed in PH patients, which might be associated with increased levels of oxidized arachidonic and linoleic acids.

It is important to note because oxidized lipids trigger an inflammatory reaction that causes DNA damage commonly observed in PAH. Also, miR-193 downregulation activates insulin growth factor 1 receptor and hence induces proliferation. Treatment with a high-density lipoprotein mimetic, 4F peptide, reversed monocrotaline and hypoxia-induced PH by blocking oxidized lipid action and restoring the levels of miR-193.(Sharma et al., 2014)

Because of the change in expression patterns of many miRNAs that modulate key pathogenic pathways in PAH, they present promising targets for development of potential therapeutics. It is not surprising that mimics and antago-miR therapies have reached clinical trials

DNA Methylation

Cytosine-phospho-guanine (CpG) islands are regions of DNA where a cytosine nucleotide occurs next to a guanine nucleotide in the linear sequence of bases along its length. They are present in gene promoter regions and methylation of cytosines leads to silencing gene expression. It was reported that superoxide dismutase 2 (SOD2) gene was downregulated in PAH via hypermethylation of CpG islands.(Archer et al., 2010) SOD2 downregulation contributes to the normoxic activation of the transcription factor HIF-1 implicated in the Warburg effect and in PAH-PASMC proliferation. It was supported by the evidence that there is an increased expression of DNA methyltransferase-1 and 3B, and the inhibition of these methyltransferases restores SOD2 expression and thus ameliorates PAH.(Archer et al., 2010) However, not much is known about methylation processes in PAH and need further investigation.

Modification of Histone Proteins

Histone acetylation and deacetylation are dynamic processes by which the lysine residues within the N-terminal tail protruding from the histone core of the nucleosome are acetylated and deacetylated. They are regulated by the balance between the enzymes histone acetyltransferases and histone deacetylases (HDACs). In the recent past, many HDAC inhibitors have been developed for their antimalignant and cardioprotective effects and several studies demonstrated that HDAC inhibitors are capable of reversing experimental PAH. For example, in a recent study, Zhao et al. demonstrated increased levels of HDAC1 and HDAC5 in IPAH lungs and that their inhibition improves PAH by decreasing the expression of prosurvival protein Bcl-2 and increasing p21 expression.(Zhao et al., 2012) It has been proposed that inhibition of class I HDACs counteracts the PDGF-induced PASMC migration and proliferation via inhibition of Akt and downregulation of cyclin D1 expression.(Galletti et al., 2014) Nonetheless, some studies showed that HDAC inhibitors might have detrimental effects on right ventricles especially by decreasing angiogenesis. Hence, the role of HDAC inhibitors in PAH is debatable.

Potential Implication of Long Noncoding RNA

Long intergenic non-coding RNA (lncRNA) are over 200 nucleotides that regulate histone modification, transcription, and posttranscriptional mechanism such as splicing and thus have become targets of interest in cardiovascular diseases and cancer. During hypoxic conditions, metastasis associated lung adenocarcinoma transcript 1 (MALAT-1) lncRNA which is expressed by ECs and regulates vessel growth is upregulated resulting in an EC pro-proliferative effect and its inhibition in vivo reduces vascular growth.(Michalik et al., 2014) Expression of lncRNA-p21, which induces the proliferation/apoptosis imbalance in vascular SMCs is decreased in neointimal hyperplasia observed in carotid injury, a model very similar to vascular remodeling in PAH. Together, lncRNAs need to be studied further as they might be implicated in PAH by regulating changes in EC and SMC phenotypes.

Vascular Stiffening in PAH: A Cause or Consequence?

To some degree or another, stiffening of the PAs, both large elastic and small resistance vessels is seen in PAH yet it is still not clear whether arterial stiffening is a cause or a consequence. However, it is evident that PA stiffening increases flow pulsatility in the pulmonary vasculature, which results in the first insult in PAH pathogenesis, the endothelial dysfunction via stimulation of proinflammatory, vasoconstrictory, and profibrogenic mediators. The disordered flow perpetuates dysfunction of distal arteries in particular and the multifaceted role of stiffening-induced EC dysfunction is characterized by a myriad of pathologic events few of which include PA hypertrophy, inflammation, endothelial to mesecnchymal transition (EndoMT), and fibrosis. Together with other microenvironmental alterations, disordered proximal-distal PA coupling also plays a critical role in increasing the ventricular afterload, ultimately resulting in RV failure and hence premature death. Due to the complex interplay of various contributing factors and multiple cell types, the molecular mechanism(s) that exacerbate vascular stiffening and hence progression of PAH, effective therapeutic targeting to cure the disease rather than treating the symptoms still remains a distant dream.(Tan, Madhavan, Hunter, Park, & Stenmark, 2014)

Other contributing factors – It has been emphasized through genetic and pathophysiologic studies that a number of mediators including prostaglandin I_2 (prostacyclin), endothelin-1, nitric oxide, angiopoietin-1, serotonin, cytokines, chemokines, and members of the transforming-growth factor-beta superfamily are involved in the initiation and progression of PAH (Humbert et al., 2004) In addition, animal and clinical studies have revealed an increase in sympathetic activity in PAH. Distension of the main pulmonary artery results in excitation of baroreceptors in or near the bifurcation of the main pulmonary artery and hence causes a significant rise in pulmonary vascular resistance. Therefore, denervation of the pulmonary vasculature presents a potential therapeutic target. (Aramendia, Taguini, Fourcade, & Taguini, 1963; Juratsch, Jengo, Castagna, & Laks, 1980; Laks, Juratsch, Garner, Beazell, & Criley, 1975; Osorio & Russek, 1962)

Treatment

Goal of treatment for PAH not only includes survival of the patients but also improving the patient's symptoms and quality of life. Assessments to measure response to treatment include improvement in exercise capacity (6 minute walk test, cardiopulmonary exercise test, and treadmill test), hemodynamics, and survival. An important aspect of PAH pathogenesis comprises of endothelial dysfunction leading to an imbalance of vasodilatory and vasoconstrictory mediators characterized by sustained reduction in vasodilatory mediators (such as PGI2 and NO), and upregulation of vasoconstrictors (such as ET-1).(Giaid & Saleh, 1995) The understanding of molecules involved in the regulation of pulmonary vasomotion has led to the development of currently approved PAH therapies, targeting one of the following key pathways: (1) prostacyclin (PGI2), (2) nitric oxide (NO), and (3) endothelin-1 (ET-1) pathways.

Basic Measures and Conventional Therapies

Exercise Rehabilitation - Deconditioning and skeletal muscle dysfunction are common in PAH. Few randomized controlled trials (RCTs) support that in patients with PAH, supervised rehabilitation helps improving exercise capacity and quality of life.

Oxygen Therapy - In patients with PAH, hypoxemia occurs at rest, during exercise, and during sleep. Sleep-disordered breathing is common in precapillary PAH and has been reported in up to two-thirds of patients with PH and an associated right heart failure. Hence, oxygen is prescribed to maintain PaO2 above 60 mm Hg.

Anticoagulation - Anticoagulation is recommended in PAH with vitamin K antagonist aiming for an international normalized ratio (INR) of 1.5 to 2.5, unless contraindicated. Because the evidence for anticoagulation in other forms of PAH is even weaker, careful risk-benefit assessment is warranted, especially in patients with systemic sclerosis who are at a higher risk for bleeding.(Henkens, Hazenoot, Boonstra, Huisman, & Vonk-Noordegraaf, 2013) Anticoagulation is also recommended for patients receiving continuous intravenous prostanoid therapy to minimize catheter-related thrombosis.

Calcium Channel Blockers - Vasoreactivity testing should only be performed with short-acting pulmonary vasodilators, and inhaled NO is currently the agent of choice based on established evidence from literature. Slow uptitration but high-maintenance dosages of calcium channel blockers, typically diltiazem, 240–720 mg; nifedipine, 120–240 mg is required. Patients who do not achieve New York heart association (NYHA) functional class (FC) I to II status and/or sustained hemodynamic response are required to be considered for other PAH therapies.

Other basic measures – A careful use of diuretics to provide symptomatic relief via reduction of right ventricular preload and improvement in left ventricular filling is still a go to option. Management of supraventricular arrhythmias is often difficult and is poorly tolerated in patients with progressive PAH. Judicious use of early electric cardioversion and antiarrhythmic drugs such as amiodarone can be considered to maintain sinus rhythm.(Olsson, Nickel, Tongers, & Hoeper, 2013) Digoxin might be useful for rate control; however, drugs with negative inotropic effects must be avoided.

Approved PAH Therapies

1) Prostacyclin Pathway

Endogenous prostaglandin 12 (PGI2), produced mainly by endothelial cells is a vasodilator, antithrombotic, anti-inflammatory, and antiproliferative agent that binds to prostaglandin I (IP) receptors with downstream effect on cAMP levels.

Epoprostenol - Intravenous (IV) epoprostenol, the first targeted therapy approved for the treatment of PAH is a prostacyclin analogue. Till date, it remains the only drug exhibiting survival benefit in randomized control trials (RCTs). However, administration of IV epoprostenol is highly complex, and must be given as a continuous infusion via an indwelling catheter which is associated with potential complications.(Doran et al., 2008) Patients and caregivers are required to be educated on appropriate catheter care to prevent catheter-related infections.

Iloprost – Iloprost can be administered via both inhaled and IV routes, although the inhaled route has only been tested in RCTs so far. To achieve clinical efficacy, inhaled iloprost must be administered at least 6 times a day as it has a very short half-life of 25 minutes.

Treprostinil – Treprostinil can be administered via the IV, subcutaneous (SC), inhaled, and oral routes as it has greater chemical stability and longer half-life than epoprostenol. Continuous SC administration of treprostinil has an added advantage as it bypasses the practical difficulties and complications associated with indwelling central venous catheters.

2) Endothelin Pathway

Endothelin-1 (ET-1) is one of the most potent vasoconstrictors that exerts its effects on two distinct receptor subtypes, ETA and ETB receptors. ETA receptor is highly localized to PASMC, while ETB receptor is predominantly expressed on the endothelium but can also be found on PASMC. Although both ETA and ETB receptors regulate smooth muscle constriction and proliferation, ETB receptor is the major isoform that is involved in the local clearance of ET-1 and induces vasodilation via the release of NO and PGI2 from endothelial cells. Apart from promoting proliferation of PAECs and

PASMCs, ET-1 is also greatly implicated in fibroblast activation, contraction, and synthesis of the extracellular matrix proteins.(Shi-Wen et al., 2001)

Bosentan – The first oral agent approved for the treatment of PAH, Bosentan, is a nonselective dual ET-1 receptor antagonist. It has also been shown to improve both exercise capacity and hemodynamics in congenital heart disease-PAH. Increase in the levels of liver transaminase is a common side effect and hence, periodic monitoring of liver function tests is mandatory in patients undergoing bosentan therapy.

Ambrisentan – Ambrisentan, a selective ETA receptor antagonist, demonstrated improved outcomes in 6MWD and NYHA FC in patients with PAH.(Galie et al., 2008) Risk of liver injury and potential for drug-drug interaction is low when compared to bosentan. However, patients should be monitored for peripheral edema, a common side effect associated with ambrisentan therapy. Interestingly, despite the theoretical advantage of selective ETA receptor blockade considering the role played by ETB receptor in local ET-1 clearance, clinical efficacy appears broadly similar between bosentan and ambrisentan.

Macitentan - Macitentan is a dual ET-1 receptor antagonist that demonstrates high lipophilicity, increased receptor affinity, and prolonged receptor binding than bosentan due to modification in the structure.(Iglarz et al., 2008) Therefore, macitentan has enhanced tissue penetration capabilities with sustained antagonism against ET-1 receptors.

3) Nitric Oxide-cGMP Pathway

Reduced NO production and bioavailability in endothelial cells is a key feature of endothelial dysfunction that initiates the pathogenesis of PAH. NO released from ECs activates soluble guanylate cyclase resulting in smooth muscle relaxation. In addition, NO is also a potent inhibitor of smooth muscle proliferation and platelet activation. This pathway is highly implicated in PAH and can be manipulated via direct administration of NO; inhibition of phosphodiesterase-5 (PDE-5), an enzyme responsible for cGMP degradation or stimulation of sGC.

Sildenafil – Phosphodiesterases (PDEs) are the enzymes that regulate the intracellular degradation of cGMP. PDE-5 plays a key role in the regulation of smooth muscle tone in the pulmonary vascular bed and the corpus cavernosum. Sildenafil, the first PDE-5 inhibitor approved for the treatment of PAH, demonstrated that the majority (60%) of patients improved or maintained their functional status at 3 years of treatment at a dose of 80 mg 3 times a day.(Rubin et al., 2011)

Tadalafil - Tadalafil is a structurally distinct PDE-5 inhibitor in comparison with sildenafil, which accounts for its different pharmacokinetic properties and longer half-life. Tadalafil is used to improve the ability to exercise in patients with PAH.

Riociguat - Riociguat is a sGC stimulator that not only maintains sGC in its active configuration when low levels of NO are available but also produces cGMP even in the absence of NO.(Stasch et al., 2001) Since there is a deficiency in endothelial NOS and, hence, NO production in patients with PAH, riociguat offers a better symptomatic relief. Riociguat and NO together have a more pronounced therapeutic effect than either of their single therapies.

New Drugs in Early Phase of Development

i) Newer Agents Targeting Established Vasodilatory Pathways

Nonprostanoid IP Receptor Agonists – Selexipag, a nonprostanoid diphenylpyrazine derivative acts on the human prostaglandin I2 (IP) receptor. It is orally available. Because it has high specificity for the IP receptor, it has an added advantage over prostacyclin analogues due to reduced theoretical side effects associated with the activation of other prostanoid receptors that mediate unwanted side effects.

Nitrite-NO Pathway - NO can be generated via an alternative NOS-independent pathway involving the anion nitrite (NO2–), in addition to the classical L-arginine-NOS-NO pathway. In a recent study, inhaled NO2– resulted in potent pulmonary vasodilatation without an effect on systemic blood pressure in an ovine model of hypoxia-induced pulmonary vasoconstriction.(Hunter et al., 2004) It has also been shown that treatment with inhaled nitrite in monocrotaline- and hypoxia-induced rodent models of PAH is effective in preventing and reversing PAH. NO2– is chemically more stable than NO and has a half-life of 30 minutes, which has implications for potential clinical translation because intermittent dosing is possible.

Inhibition of Cyclic Nucleotides Metabolism - The cyclic nucleotides cGMP and cAMP are greatly involved in regulating vasomotor tone and vascular smooth muscle proliferation. Apart from PDE mediated degradation, intracellular cyclic nucleotide levels are also regulated by an active efflux transport system. A member of the ATP-binding cassette transporter family, multidrug resistance–associated protein 4 (MRP4), mediates the cellular efflux of cyclic nucleotides, and the transport of other endogenous metabolites as well as drugs. Recently, it was found that MRP4 is overexpressed in the pulmonary arteries from PAH patients and also in mice exposed to hypoxia. In mice, administration of a MRP4 inhibitor, MK571 reversed hypoxia-induced PAH. Supporting this, recent data showed that MPR4 knockout mice are protected from hypoxia-induced pulmonary vascular remodeling and also display reduced inflammatory cell recruitment to pulmonary arteries. Together, these observations suggest that inhibition of MRP4 might represent an interesting target for human PAH.

ii) Tyrosine Kinase Inhibition

The pro-proliferative and antiapoptotic phenotypic characteristic of PAH vasculopathy has led to an interest in the role of growth factors in PAH.

Imatinib - Imatinib is a nonspecific tyrosine kinase inhibitor (TKI) which targets the bcr-abl fusion protein, PDGFR, and c-kit.(Table 1) Imatinib improved pulmonary hemodynamics in a subgroup of patients with severe PAH in a small phase II study and hence led to a larger phase III study which showed outcomes favoring imatinib group.(Ghofrani et al., 2010) However, because of the differential dropout rate and no improvements in NYHA FC or time to clinical worsening, it is difficult to interpret the efficacy of the drug. In addition to that, treatment with imatinib was poorly tolerated among patients with PAH and serious adverse events were common including the occurrence of subdural hematomas. There is a risk of cardiotoxicity with the use of TKIs, and hence requires further investigation.

iii) Serotonin System

Serotonin induces pulmonary artery vasoconstriction and PASMC proliferation. In IPAH, it was reported that there is a depletion of platelet storage of serotonin, elevation of peripheral blood serotonin levels, enhanced serotonin transporter expression and increased proliferation in response to serotonin stimulation by PASMCs. However, a phase II study of terguride, a 5HT-2 receptor antagonist, has shown that it was not associated with any improvements in either hemodynamics or exercise capacity as opposed to the expected improved outcomes.

Table 1. Drugs under investigation for potential use in the treatment of pulmonary hypertension

Investigational Compound	Class	Mechanism of action	Stage of development
Vasoactive intestinal peptide	Vasodilator	Relaxes the vasculature and reduces the effects of vasoconstrictors	Clinical trials
eNOS co-factor sapropterin dihydrochloride	Endothelial NO synthase couplers	Dimerizes/couples with eNOS in order to produce NO and to cease production of vasoconstrictors such as superoxide	Clinical trials
Fasudil	Rho Kinase inhibitor	Regulates intracellular calcium levels and hence causes vasodilation	Clinical trials
Terguride	Serotonin receptor antagonist	Inhibits the vasoconstrictive and mitogenic properties of serotonin	Clinical trials
Apelin	Vasodilatory peptide	Vasodilatory effects and reduces pulmonary arterial pressure	Pre-clinical studies
Tocilizumab	Anti-IL6 monoclonal antibody	Immunosuppression	Pre-clinical studies
Rapamycin	Immunosuppressant	Antiproliferative agent	Pre-clinical studies
Gefitinib, Erlotinib and Lapatinib	EGF receptor antagonists	Inhibit EGF-induced smooth muscle cell proliferation	Pre-clinical studies
Rosiglitazone	PPARγ agonist	Forms a complex with β-catenin appears to trigger the transcription on apelin, a vasodilator	Pre-clinical studies
Dichloroacetate	Pyruvate dehydrogenase kinase (PDK) inhibitor	Decreases proliferation and increases apoptosis of PASMCs	Pre-clinical studies
Imatinib	Tyrosine kinase Inhibitor	Targets Bcr-Abl fusion protein, PDGFR, c-kit	Clinical trials

Table 1. (Continued)

Investigational Compound	Class	Mechanism of action	Stage of development
Simvastatin	Statin	Indirectly blocks the posttranslational isoprenylation and activation of Rho and Ras small GT Pases, increase endothelial NO production	Pre-clinical studies
Selexipag	Nonprostanoid IP Receptor Agonist	Acts on prostaglandin I2 (IP) receptor and causes vasodilation	Pre-clinical studies

iv) Vasoactive Intestinal Peptide

Vasoactive intestinal peptide that mediates smooth muscle relaxation via activation of adenylate cyclase and generation of cAMP was originally discovered in gut and consists of 28 amino acids. Despite initial reports of hemodynamic and functional improvements in small uncontrolled studies,(Leuchte et al., 2008) a phase II RCT of inhaled vasoactive intestinal peptide in PAH patients was unable to demonstrate any beneficial effects both in hemodynamics or exercise capacity. A thorough investigation on the mechanism of action and efficacy of the peptide should be carried out before proceeding to larger clinical trials.

v) RhoA/Rho-Kinase Signaling Pathway

The RhoA/ROCK signaling pathway is activated in the pulmonary arteries of PAH, and ROCK can lead to smooth muscle hypercontractility by suppressing myosin phosphatase activity which controls Ca2+ sensitivity of myofilaments. Fasudil, a potent specific ROCK inhibitor demonstrated a 17% reduction in PVR in a small observational study involving patients with severe PAH upon IV administration of the drug.(Fukumoto et al., 2005)

vi) Statins

Statins exhibit a wide range of cholesterol-independent pleiotropic properties including antiproliferative, anti-inflammatory, and antithrombotic effects. Also, statins indirectly block the posttranslational isoprenylation and activation of Rho and Ras small GTPases, increase endothelial NO production, and also enhance the expression of BMPR-II in experimental PAH (Table 1). It has been recently shown that simvastatin therapy was associated with a small but significant reduction in right ventricular mass at 6 months, but this effect was not sustained at 12 months.(Wilkins et al., 2010)

vii) Apelin

Apelin, an endogenous peptide exerts vasodilatory effects on the pulmonary vasculature and it is in part associated with the regulation of endothelial NOS levels. Apelin has been identified as a key downstream target of BMPR-II signaling where its expression is controlled by BMPR-II signaling mediated by a complex between β-catenin and peroxisome proliferator–activated receptor gamma.(Alastalo et al., 2011) Apelin is being investigated for its potential as a therapeutic target of PAH in experimental and clinical studies. (Table 1)

viii) Anti-inflammatory therapies

Efficacy of anti-inflammatory therapies has been explored mostly in connective tissue disorder-PAH, and small case series have reported the clinical response to immunosuppression when a combination of cyclophosphamide with glucocorticoids was used. (Table 1) However, beneficial effects appear restricted to PAH associated with lupus and mixed connective tissue disorders rather than systemic sclerosis–associated PAH.

ix) Restoration of BMPR-II Signaling Axis

Ataluren - Ataluren interacts with ribosomes to enable the read through of premature stop codons. It is a phase III investigational drug in clinical trials for cystic fibrosis. A recent study demonstrated that treatment with ataluren restores BMPR-II expression in peripheral blood and lung vascular cells from patients carrying nonsense BMPR-2 mutations.(Drake, Dunmore, McNelly, Morrell, & Aldred, 2013)

Antagomirs - Micro-RNAs (miR) are small noncoding RNA molecules containing about 22 nucleotides that regulate gene expression at the post-transcriptional level. MiR-17/92 cluster, mainly miR-20a exerts negative regulatory effects on BMPR-II expression via an interleukin-6–dependent STAT3 pathway. Antagomirs, a novel class of chemically engineered oligonucleotides can silencince miRs. In the hypoxia-induced mouse model of PAH, treatment with the antagomir directed against miR-20a enhanced the expression of BMPR-II in lung tissues and attenuated pulmonary vascular remodeling.(Brock et al., 2014)

Tacrolimus - FK506 (tacrolimus), a calcineurin inhibitor was recently found to be a candidate compound that can upregulate BMPR-II signaling. Normal signal transduction involves BMPR-II forming a heterodimer complex with sister type-1 BMP receptors. In the presence of ligand binding, BMPR-II phosphorylates the intracellular domain of type-1 receptors, leading to activation of cytosolic Smad signaling cascade. FKBP12 is a molecule that interacts with type-1 BMP receptors and blocks its activation by occupying the phosphorylation site. FK506 binds to and removes FKBP12 from type-1 BMP receptors, restoring normal signaling.(Spiekerkoetter et al., 2013) It has been shown that treatment with low-dose of FK506 reverses both monocrotaline-induced and hypoxia/Sugen–induced PAH in rats.

Procedures/Nonmedical Therapies

Lung Transplantation - Despite targeted PAH therapy, lung transplantation remains a destination therapy for most PAH patients. Considering limited organ availability and high mortality rates of PAH patients awaiting transplantation, eligible patients for whom first-line treatment strategies have failed should be immediately referred for transplantation assessment. Although double-lung transplantation is the preferred option for PAH, heart-lung transplantation remains necessary for some patients and is adopted for patients with refractory right heart failure.(Fadel et al., 2010)

Atrial Septostomy and Potts Shunt - Balloon atrial septostomy is a procedure which creates artificial right-to-left shunt to decompress the right ventricle as there is an excessive right ventricular hypertrophy in patients with progressive PAH. It can be accomplished percutaneously with careful graded balloon dilation and can improve peripheral oxygen delivery despite a fall in systemic arterial saturation because of a compensatory rise in cardiac output.(Kurzyna et al., 2007) Atrial septostomy is not a highly recommended procedure because it is associated with high periprocedural mortality in patients with markedly elevated right atrial pressure and should only be considered as a palliative therapy or bridge to transplantation in centers with experience in this procedure.

An alternative method of right ventricular decompression is the Potts shunt which involves creation of an anastomosis between the descending aorta and left pulmonary artery. In the setting of suprasystemic pulmonary artery pressure, Potts shunt has a theoretical advantage over septostomy which is the sparing of the cerebral and coronary circulation from deoxygenated blood. Interestingly, a small case series of adults with NYHA FC IV PAH demonstrated the feasibility of the creation of Potts shunt via a minimally invasive percutaneous approach.(Esch et al., 2013) However, further investigation is required to assess the safety and efficacy of this innovative technique.

Pulmonary Artery Denervation –A recently emerging novel nonmedical therapy for PAH, pulmonary artery denervation involves borrowing the concept of renal artery denervation. The presumed mechanism of action of this technique is via the abolishment of sympathetic nerve supply to the pulmonary circulation. In a recent first-in-human single-center study, 13 patients underwent pulmonary artery denervation with the use of a dedicated radiofrequency ablation catheter resulting in significant reduction of mean PAP and improvement in 6MWT. However, these preliminary results require further confirmation, because the negative findings from a trial of renal denervation for resistant hypertension serves as a cautionary reminder that device-based therapies must be subjected to rigorous evaluation before adoption into clinical practice.

Recent understanding on left ventricular failure suggests alterations in electromechanical coupling and hemodynamics that have responded dramatically to cardiac resynchronization therapy. Given the similarities between RV and LV remodeling in response to dyssynchrony, it is reasonable to investigate the possibility of resynchronization therapy for the failing RV. Multiple studies including animals, a computer simulation analysis, and one study involving patients with chronic thromboembolic pulmonary hypertension have shown acute improvements in cardiac function and hemodynamics with RV pacing. However, it is too soon to conclude the efficiency of this technique yet as it is not clear if these promising results would apply to other types of pulmonary hypertension, Further investigation is required to determine whether resynchronization therapy for RV failure in patients with PAH will become a viable treatment option.(Rasmussen, Thenappan, Benditt, Weir, & Pritzker, 2014)

Expected Novel Drugs in Future/ Therapies under Investigation

Although vasoconstriction remains a major component of the pathophysiology of PAH, there has been a growing curiosity in the past few years not only for agents which act as vasodilators, but also for those with antiproliferative and antiremodeling effects. There is accumulating evidence that the pulmonary vasculopathy is related to inflammation and a proproliferative/antiapoptotic phenotype of pulmonary artery smooth muscle cells. Of note, PAH is associated with few of the hallmark characteristics of cancer, hence opening the way to new therapeutic strategies developed in oncology. (Paulin, Courboulin, Barrier, & Bonnet, 2011) In a preclinical study, Cai et al., showed that a phenoxybutanoic acid derivative, 6e was effective in relieving hypoxia-induced pulmonary arterial hypertension and right ventricular weight ratio compared to another derivative 6g and a reference compound BQ123. Therefore, 6e may have potential for further development as a therapeutic agent for the treatment of cardiovascular diseases.(Cai et al., 2015) Several miRNAs are under preclinical and clinical investigation to evaluate their potential for PAH treatment. Several Warburg effect inhibitors such as dichloroacetate (PDH kinase inhibitor) and NFAT inhibitors, show promising pharmacological effects for PAH treatment, and are in ongoing clinical studies in PAH.

Gap in Knowledge

Although drug therapies have significantly improved symptoms, hemodynamics and exercise capacity in patients with PAH, (Galie et al., 2005; Rubin et al., 2002) the molecular mechanisms of PAH, a disease for which there is no cure, is not yet fully understood. There is remarkable evidence that the endothelial dysfunction is a key factor in triggering vasoconstriction and subsequent vascular remodeling. However, PAH pathobiology is highly complex and involves many components such as proproliferative and antiapoptotic PAECs and PASMCs, a proinflammatory environment, and epigenetic deregulation. Together, these lead to an increased pulmonary vascular wall thickness, muscularization of small arterioles, and formation of PLs observed in PAH. The underlying molecular mechanisms that trigger the phenotypic switch of endothelial and smooth muscle cells in the pulmonary vasculature still remains unclear. A thorough understanding of PAH pathophysiology from adaptation to remodeling of the PAs will be instrumental in developing new therapeutic strategies for treating the disease rather than the symptoms. Unraveling the causes of proximal vascular stiffening as well as those of HPF-induced cellular and molecular alterations in the distal pulmonary vasculatures, could lead to important new therapeutic options to halt PA remodeling and PH progression. Further refining a mimetic vascular physiological model similar to the so-called lung on a chip may be instrumental to such understanding. Future studies should be aimed at the root cause of arterial stiffening to develop therapeutic interventions which will treat the cause of the disease and not the symptoms.(Tan et al., 2014)

References

Abe, K., Toba, M., Alzoubi, A., Ito, M., Fagan, K. A., Cool, C. D., . . . Oka, M. (2010). Formation of plexiform lesions in experimental severe pulmonary arterial hypertension. *Circulation*, *121*(25), 2747-2754. doi: 10.1161/CIRCULATIONAHA.109.927681

Alastalo, T. P., Li, M., Perez Vde, J., Pham, D., Sawada, H., Wang, J. K., . . . Rabinovitch, M. (2011). Disruption of PPARgamma/beta-catenin-mediated regulation of apelin impairs BMP-induced mouse and human pulmonary arterial EC survival. *J Clin Invest*, *121*(9), 3735-3746. doi: 10.1172/JCI43382

Aramendia, P., Taguini, C. M., Fourcade, A. & Taguini, A. C. (1963). Reflex Vasomotor Activity during Unilateral Occlusion of the Pulmonary Artery. *Am Heart J*, *66*, 53-60.

Archer, S. L., Marsboom, G., Kim, G. H., Zhang, H. J., Toth, P. T., Svensson, E. C., . . . Rehman, J. (2010). Epigenetic attenuation of mitochondrial superoxide dismutase 2 in pulmonary arterial hypertension: a basis for excessive cell proliferation and a new therapeutic target. *Circulation, 121*(24), 2661-2671. doi: 10.1161/CIRCULATIONAHA.109.916098

Austin, E. D. & Loyd, J. E. (2014). The genetics of pulmonary arterial hypertension. *Circ Res, 115*(1), 189-202. doi: 10.1161/CIRCRESAHA.115.303404

Badesch, D. B., Raskob, G. E., Elliott, C. G., Krichman, A. M., Farber, H. W., Frost, A. E., . . . McGoon, M. D. (2010). Pulmonary arterial hypertension: baseline characteristics from the REVEAL Registry. *Chest, 137*(2), 376-387. doi: 10.1378/chest.09-1140

Barst, R. J., McGoon, M., Torbicki, A., Sitbon, O., Krowka, M. J., Olschewski, H. & Gaine, S. (2004). Diagnosis and differential assessment of pulmonary arterial hypertension. *J Am Coll Cardiol, 43*(12 Suppl S), 40S-47S. doi: 10.1016/j.jacc.2004.02.032

Bertero, T., Lu, Y., Annis, S., Hale, A., Bhat, B., Saggar, R., . . . Chan, S. Y. (2014). Systems-level regulation of microRNA networks by miR-130/301 promotes pulmonary hypertension. *J Clin Invest, 124*(8), 3514-3528. doi: 10.1172/JCI74773

Bienertova-Vasku, J., Novak, J. & Vasku, A. (2014). MicroRNAs in pulmonary arterial hypertension: pathogenesis, diagnosis and treatment. *J Am Soc Hypertens*. doi: 10.1016/j.jash.2014.12.011

Brock, M., Samillan, V. J., Trenkmann, M., Schwarzwald, C., Ulrich, S., Gay, R. E., . . . Huber, L. C. (2014). AntagomiR directed against miR-20a restores functional BMPR2 signalling and prevents vascular remodelling in hypoxia-induced pulmonary hypertension. *Eur Heart J, 35*(45), 3203-3211. doi: 10.1093/eurheartj/ehs060

Cai, J., Liu, L., Hong, K. H., Wang, P., Li, L., Cao, M., . . . Ji, M. (2015). Discovery of phenoxybutanoic acid derivatives as potent endothelin antagonists with antihypertensive activity. *Bioorg Med Chem*. doi: 10.1016/j.bmc.2015.01.003

Caruso, P., Dempsie, Y., Stevens, H. C., McDonald, R. A., Long, L., Lu, R., . . . Baker, A. H. (2012). A role for miR-145 in pulmonary arterial hypertension: evidence from mouse models and patient samples. *Circ Res, 111*(3), 290-300. doi: 10.1161/CIRCRESAHA.112.267591

Choi, E. Y., Jin, J. Y., Lee, J. Y., Choi, J. I., Choi, I. S. & Kim, S. J. (2011). Melatonin inhibits Prevotella intermedia lipopolysaccharide-induced production of nitric oxide and interleukin-6 in murine macrophages by suppressing NF-kappaB and STAT1 activity. *J Pineal Res, 50*(2), 197-206. doi: 10.1111/j.1600-079X.2010.00829.x

Christman, B. W., McPherson, C. D., Newman, J. H., King, G. A., Bernard, G. R., Groves, B. M. & Loyd, J. E. (1992). An imbalance between the excretion of thromboxane and prostacyclin metabolites in pulmonary hypertension. *N Engl J Med, 327*(2), 70-75. doi: 10.1056/NEJM199207093270202

Cottrill, K. A. & Chan, S. Y. (2013). Metabolic dysfunction in pulmonary hypertension: the expanding relevance of the Warburg effect. *Eur J Clin Invest, 43*(8), 855-865. doi: 10.1111/eci.12104

Courboulin, A., Paulin, R., Giguere, N. J., Saksouk, N., Perreault, T., Meloche, J., . . . Bonnet, S. (2011). Role for miR-204 in human pulmonary arterial hypertension. *J Exp Med, 208*(3), 535-548. doi: 10.1084/jem.20101812

Crosswhite, P., Chen, K. & Sun, Z. (2014). AAV delivery of tumor necrosis factor-alpha short hairpin RNA attenuates cold-induced pulmonary hypertension and pulmonary arterial remodeling. *Hypertension, 64*(5), 1141-1150. doi: 10.1161/HYPERTENSIONAHA.114.03791

Cuttica, M. J., Langenickel, T., Noguchi, A., Machado, R. F., Gladwin, M. T. & Boehm, M. (2011). Perivascular T-cell infiltration leads to sustained pulmonary artery remodeling after endothelial cell damage. *Am J Respir Cell Mol Biol, 45*(1), 62-71. doi: 10.1165/rcmb.2009-0365OC

Doran, A. K., Ivy, D. D., Barst, R. J., Hill, N., Murali, S., Benza, R. L. & Scientific Leadership Council of the Pulmonary Hypertension, A. (2008). Guidelines for the prevention of central venous catheter-related blood stream infections with prostanoid therapy for pulmonary arterial hypertension. *Int J Clin Pract Suppl*(160), 5-9. doi: 10.1111/j.1742-1241.2008.01811.x

Drake, K. M., Dunmore, B. J., McNelly, L. N., Morrell, N. W. & Aldred, M. A. (2013). Correction of nonsense BMPR2 and SMAD9 mutations by ataluren in pulmonary arterial hypertension. *Am J Respir Cell Mol Biol, 49*(3), 403-409. doi: 10.1165/rcmb.2013-0100OC

Esch, J. J., Shah, P. B., Cockrill, B. A., Farber, H. W., Landzberg, M. J., Mehra, M. R., . . . Marshall, A. C. (2013). Transcatheter Potts shunt creation in patients with severe pulmonary arterial hypertension: initial clinical experience. *J Heart Lung Transplant, 32*(4), 381-387. doi: 10.1016/j.healun.2013.01.1049

Fadel, E., Mercier, O., Mussot, S., Leroy-Ladurie, F., Cerrina, J., Chapelier, A., . . . Dartevelle, P. (2010). Long-term outcome of double-lung and heart-lung transplantation for pulmonary hypertension: a comparative retrospective study of 219 patients. *Eur J Cardiothorac Surg, 38*(3), 277-284. doi: 10.1016/j.ejcts.2010.02.039

Farber, H. W. & Loscalzo, J. (2004). Pulmonary arterial hypertension. *N Engl J Med, 351*(16), 1655-1665. doi: 10.1056/NEJMra035488

Fukumoto, Y., Matoba, T., Ito, A., Tanaka, H., Kishi, T., Hayashidani, S., . . . Shimokawa, H. (2005). Acute vasodilator effects of a Rho-kinase inhibitor, fasudil, in patients with severe pulmonary hypertension. *Heart, 91*(3), 391-392. doi: 10.1136/hrt.2003.029470

Galie, N., Ghofrani, H. A., Torbicki, A., Barst, R. J., Rubin, L. J., Badesch, D., . . . Sildenafil Use in Pulmonary Arterial Hypertension Study, G. (2005). Sildenafil citrate therapy for pulmonary arterial hypertension. *N Engl J Med, 353*(20), 2148-2157. doi: 10.1056/NEJMoa050010

Galie, N., Hoeper, M. M., Humbert, M., Torbicki, A., Vachiery, J. L., Barbera, J. A., . . . Guidelines, E. S. C. C. f. P. (2009). Guidelines for the diagnosis and treatment of pulmonary hypertension: the Task Force for the Diagnosis and Treatment of Pulmonary Hypertension of the European Society of Cardiology (ESC) and the European Respiratory Society (ERS), endorsed by the International Society of Heart and Lung Transplantation (ISHLT). *Eur Heart J, 30*(20), 2493-2537. doi: 10.1093/eurheartj/ehp297

Galie, N., Olschewski, H., Oudiz, R. J., Torres, F., Frost, A., Ghofrani, H. A., . . . Ambrisentan in Pulmonary Arterial Hypertension, R. D.-B. P.-C. M. E. S. G. (2008). Ambrisentan for the treatment of pulmonary arterial hypertension: results of the ambrisentan in pulmonary arterial hypertension, randomized, double-blind, placebo-controlled, multicenter, efficacy (ARIES) study 1 and 2. *Circulation, 117*(23), 3010-3019. doi: 10.1161/CIRCULATIONAHA.107.742510

Galletti, M., Cantoni, S., Zambelli, F., Valente, S., Palazzini, M., Manes, A., . . . Ventura, C. (2014). Dissecting histone deacetylase role in pulmonary arterial smooth muscle cell proliferation and migration. *Biochem Pharmacol, 91*(2), 181-190. doi: 10.1016/j.bcp.2014.07.011

Ghofrani, H. A., Morrell, N. W., Hoeper, M. M., Olschewski, H., Peacock, A. J., Barst, R. J., . . . Pascoe, S. (2010). Imatinib in pulmonary arterial hypertension patients with inadequate response to established therapy. *Am J Respir Crit Care Med, 182*(9), 1171-1177. doi: 10.1164/rccm.201001-0123OC

Giaid, A. & Saleh, D. (1995). Reduced expression of endothelial nitric oxide synthase in the lungs of patients with pulmonary hypertension. *N Engl J Med, 333*(4), 214-221. doi: 10.1056/NEJM199507273330403

Giaid, A., Yanagisawa, M., Langleben, D., Michel, R. P., Levy, R., Shennib, H., . . . Stewart, D. J. (1993). Expression of endothelin-1 in the lungs of patients with pulmonary hypertension. *N Engl J Med*, *328*(24), 1732-1739. doi: 10.1056/NEJM199306173282402

Goerke, S. M., Kiefer, L. S., Stark, G. B., Simunovic, F. & Finkenzeller, G. (2014). mir-126 modulates angiogenic growth parameters of peripheral blood endothelial progenitor cells. *Biol Chem*. doi: 10.1515/hsz-2014-0259

Guignabert, C., Alvira, C. M., Alastalo, T. P., Sawada, H., Hansmann, G., Zhao, M., . . . Rabinovitch, M. (2009). Tie2-mediated loss of peroxisome proliferator-activated receptor-gamma in mice causes PDGF receptor-beta-dependent pulmonary arterial muscularization. *Am J Physiol Lung Cell Mol Physiol*, *297*(6), L1082-1090. doi: 10.1152/ajplung.00199.2009

Henkens, I. R., Hazenoot, T., Boonstra, A., Huisman, M. V. & Vonk-Noordegraaf, A. (2013). Major bleeding with vitamin K antagonist anticoagulants in pulmonary hypertension. *Eur Respir J*, *41*(4), 872-878. doi: 10.1183/09031936.00039212

Hoeper, M. M., Bogaard, H. J., Condliffe, R., Frantz, R., Khanna, D., Kurzyna, M., . . . Badesch, D. B. (2013). Definitions and diagnosis of pulmonary hypertension. *J Am Coll Cardiol*, *62*(25 Suppl), D42-50. doi: 10.1016/j.jacc.2013.10.032

Hoeper, M. M., Huscher, D., Ghofrani, H. A., Delcroix, M., Distler, O., Schweiger, C., . . . Pittrow, D. (2013). Elderly patients diagnosed with idiopathic pulmonary arterial hypertension: results from the COMPERA registry. *Int J Cardiol*, *168*(2), 871-880. doi: 10.1016/j.ijcard.2012.10.026

Humbert, M., Morrell, N. W., Archer, S. L., Stenmark, K. R., MacLean, M. R., Lang, I. M., . . . Rabinovitch, M. (2004). Cellular and molecular pathobiology of pulmonary arterial hypertension. *J Am Coll Cardiol*, *43*(12 Suppl S), 13S-24S. doi: 10.1016/j.jacc.2004.02.029

Hunter, C. J., Dejam, A., Blood, A. B., Shields, H., Kim-Shapiro, D. B., Machado, R. F., . . . Gladwin, M. T. (2004). Inhaled nebulized nitrite is a hypoxia-sensitive NO-dependent selective pulmonary vasodilator. *Nat Med*, *10*(10), 1122-1127. doi: 10.1038/nm1109

Iglarz, M., Binkert, C., Morrison, K., Fischli, W., Gatfield, J., Treiber, A., . . . Clozel, M. (2008). Pharmacology of macitentan, an orally active tissue-targeting dual endothelin receptor antagonist. *J Pharmacol Exp Ther*, *327*(3), 736-745. doi: 10.1124/jpet.108.142976

Juratsch, C. E., Jengo, J. A., Castagna, J. & Laks, M. M. (1980). Experimental pulmonary hypertension produced by surgical and chemical denervation of the pulmonary vasculature. *Chest*, *77*(4), 525-530.

Kurzyna, M., Dabrowski, M., Bielecki, D., Fijalkowska, A., Pruszczyk, P., Opolski, G., . . . Torbicki, A. (2007). Atrial septostomy in treatment of end-stage right heart failure in patients with pulmonary hypertension. *Chest, 131*(4), 977-983. doi: 10.1378/chest.06-1227

Laks, M. M., Juratsch, C. E., Garner, D., Beazell, J. & Criley, J. M. (1975). Acute pulmonary artery hypertension produced by distention of the main pulmonary artery in the conscious dog. *Chest, 68*(6), 807-813.

Lannan, K. L., Phipps, R. P. & White, R. J. (2014). Thrombosis, platelets, microparticles and PAH: more than a clot. *Drug Discov Today, 19*(8), 1230-1235. doi: 10.1016/j.drudis.2014.04.001

Leuchte, H. H., Baezner, C., Baumgartner, R. A., Bevec, D., Bacher, G., Neurohr, C. & Behr, J. (2008). Inhalation of vasoactive intestinal peptide in pulmonary hypertension. *Eur Respir J, 32*(5), 1289-1294. doi: 10.1183/09031936.00050008

Li, M., Liu, Y., Jin, F., Sun, X., Li, Z., Liu, Y., . . . Jiang, X. (2012). Endothelin-1 induces hypoxia inducible factor 1alpha expression in pulmonary artery smooth muscle cells. *FEBS Lett, 586*(21), 3888-3893. doi: 10.1016/j.febslet.2012.08.036

Looper, K. J., Pierre, A., Dunkley, D. M., Sigal, J. J. & Langleben, D. (2009). Depressive symptoms in relation to physical functioning in pulmonary hypertension. *J Psychosom Res, 66*(3), 221-225. doi: 10.1016/ j.jpsychores.2008.09.014

Lowe, B., Grafe, K., Ufer, C., Kroenke, K., Grunig, E., Herzog, W. & Borst, M. M. (2004). Anxiety and depression in patients with pulmonary hypertension. *Psychosom Med, 66*(6), 831-836. doi: 10.1097/ 01.psy.0000145593.37594.39

Ma, J., Zhang, L., Han, W., Shen, T., Ma, C., Liu, Y., . . . Zhu, D. (2012). Activation of JNK/c-Jun is required for the proliferation, survival, and angiogenesis induced by EET in pulmonary artery endothelial cells. *J Lipid Res, 53*(6), 1093-1105. doi: 10.1194/jlr.M024398

Matura, L. A., Ventetuolo, C. E., Palevsky, H. I., Lederer, D. J., Horn, E. M., Mathai, S. C., . . . Kawut, S. M. (2015). Interleukin-6 and Tumor Necrosis Factor-Alpha Are Associated with Quality of Life-related Symptoms in Pulmonary Arterial Hypertension. *Ann Am Thorac Soc*. doi: 10.1513/AnnalsATS.201410-463OC

McGoon, M., Gutterman, D., Steen, V., Barst, R., McCrory, D. C., Fortin, T. A., . . . American College of Chest, P. (2004). Screening, early detection, and diagnosis of pulmonary arterial hypertension: ACCP evidence-based clinical practice guidelines. *Chest*, *126*(1 Suppl), 14S-34S. doi: 10.1378/chest.126.1_suppl.14S

McLaughlin, V. V., Archer, S. L., Badesch, D. B., Barst, R. J., Farber, H. W., Lindner, J. R., . . . Pulmonary Hypertension, A. (2009). ACCF/AHA 2009 expert consensus document on pulmonary hypertension a report of the American College of Cardiology Foundation Task Force on Expert Consensus Documents and the American Heart Association developed in collaboration with the American College of Chest Physicians; American Thoracic Society, Inc.; and the Pulmonary Hypertension Association. *J Am Coll Cardiol*, *53*(17), 1573-1619. doi: 10.1016/j.jacc.2009.01.004

Michalik, K. M., You, X., Manavski, Y., Doddaballapur, A., Zornig, M., Braun, T., . . . Dimmeler, S. (2014). Long noncoding RNA MALAT1 regulates endothelial cell function and vessel growth. *Circ Res*, *114*(9), 1389-1397. doi: 10.1161/CIRCRESAHA.114.303265

Montani, D., Gunther, S., Dorfmuller, P., Perros, F., Girerd, B., Garcia, G., . . . Sitbon, O. (2013). Pulmonary arterial hypertension. *Orphanet J Rare Dis*, *8*, 97. doi: 10.1186/1750-1172-8-97

Newby, A. C. (2006). Matrix metalloproteinases regulate migration, proliferation, and death of vascular smooth muscle cells by degrading matrix and non-matrix substrates. *Cardiovasc Res*, *69*(3), 614-624. doi: 10.1016/j.cardiores.2005.08.002

Olsson, K. M., Nickel, N. P., Tongers, J. & Hoeper, M. M. (2013). Atrial flutter and fibrillation in patients with pulmonary hypertension. *Int J Cardiol*, *167*(5), 2300-2305. doi: 10.1016/j.ijcard.2012.06.024

Osorio, J. & Russek, M. (1962). Reflex changes on the pulmonary and systemic pressures elicited by stimulation of baroreceptors in the pulmonary artery. *Circ Res*, *10*, 664-667.

Parikh, V. N., Jin, R. C., Rabello, S., Gulbahce, N., White, K., Hale, A., . . . Chan, S. Y. (2012). MicroRNA-21 integrates pathogenic signaling to control pulmonary hypertension: results of a network bioinformatics approach. *Circulation*, *125*(12), 1520-1532. doi: 10.1161/CIRCULATIONAHA.111.060269

Paulin, R., Courboulin, A., Barrier, M. & Bonnet, S. (2011). From oncoproteins/tumor suppressors to microRNAs, the newest therapeutic targets for pulmonary arterial hypertension. *J Mol Med (Berl)*, *89*(11), 1089-1101. doi: 10.1007/s00109-011-0788-5

Potus, F., Malenfant, S., Graydon, C., Mainguy, V., Tremblay, E., Breuils-Bonnet, S., . . . Provencher, S. (2014). Impaired angiogenesis and peripheral muscle microcirculation loss contribute to exercise intolerance in pulmonary arterial hypertension. *Am J Respir Crit Care Med*, *190*(3), 318-328. doi: 10.1164/rccm.201402-0383OC

Rasmussen, J. T., Thenappan, T., Benditt, D. G., Weir, E. K. & Pritzker, M. R. (2014). Is cardiac resynchronization therapy for right ventricular failure in pulmonary arterial hypertension of benefit? *Pulm Circ*, *4*(4), 552-559. doi: 10.1086/678470

Rosanio, S., Pelliccia, F., Gaudio, C., Greco, C., Keylani, A. M. & D'Agostino, D. C. (2014). Pulmonary arterial hypertension in adults: novel drugs and catheter ablation techniques show promise? Systematic review on pharmacotherapy and interventional strategies. *Biomed Res Int*, *2014*, 743868. doi: 10.1155/2014/743868

Rubens, C., Ewert, R., Halank, M., Wensel, R., Orzechowski, H. D., Schultheiss, H. P. & Hoeffken, G. (2001). Big endothelin-1 and endothelin-1 plasma levels are correlated with the severity of primary pulmonary hypertension. *Chest*, *120*(5), 1562-1569.

Rubin, L. J., Badesch, D. B., Barst, R. J., Galie, N., Black, C. M., Keogh, A., . . . Simonneau, G. (2002). Bosentan therapy for pulmonary arterial hypertension. *N Engl J Med*, *346*(12), 896-903. doi: 10.1056/NEJMoa012212

Rubin, L. J., Badesch, D. B., Fleming, T. R., Galie, N., Simonneau, G., Ghofrani, H. A., . . . Group, S.-S. (2011). Long-term treatment with sildenafil citrate in pulmonary arterial hypertension: the SUPER-2 study. *Chest*, *140*(5), 1274-1283. doi: 10.1378/chest.10-0969

Satoh, K., Satoh, T., Kikuchi, N., Omura, J., Kurosawa, R., Suzuki, K., . . . Shimokawa, H. (2014). Basigin mediates pulmonary hypertension by promoting inflammation and vascular smooth muscle cell proliferation. *Circ Res*, *115*(8), 738-750. doi: 10.1161/CIRCRESAHA.115.304563

Sharma, S., Umar, S., Potus, F., Iorga, A., Wong, G., Meriwether, D., . . . Eghbali, M. (2014). Apolipoprotein A-I mimetic peptide 4F rescues pulmonary hypertension by inducing microRNA-193-3p. *Circulation*, *130*(9), 776-785. doi: 10.1161/CIRCULATIONAHA.114.007405

Shi-Wen, X., Denton, C. P., Dashwood, M. R., Holmes, A. M., Bou-Gharios, G., Pearson, J. D., . . . Abraham, D. J. (2001). Fibroblast matrix gene expression and connective tissue remodeling: role of endothelin-1. *J Invest Dermatol*, *116*(3), 417-425. doi: 10.1046/j.1523-1747.2001.01256.x

Sitbon, O., Humbert, M., Jais, X., Ioos, V., Hamid, A. M., Provencher, S., . . . Simonneau, G. (2005). Long-term response to calcium channel blockers in idiopathic pulmonary arterial hypertension. *Circulation*, *111*(23), 3105-3111. doi: 10.1161/CIRCULATIONAHA.104.488486

Spiekerkoetter, E., Tian, X., Cai, J., Hopper, R. K., Sudheendra, D., Li, C. G., . . . Rabinovitch, M. (2013). FK506 activates BMPR2, rescues endothelial dysfunction, and reverses pulmonary hypertension. *J Clin Invest*, *123*(8), 3600-3613. doi: 10.1172/JCI65592

Stacher, E., Graham, B. B., Hunt, J. M., Gandjeva, A., Groshong, S. D., McLaughlin, V. V., . . . Tuder, R. M. (2012). Modern age pathology of pulmonary arterial hypertension. *Am J Respir Crit Care Med*, *186*(3), 261-272. doi: 10.1164/rccm.201201-0164OC

Staniszewska-Slezak, E., Fedorowicz, A., Kramkowski, K., Leszczynska, A., Chlopicki, S., Baranska, M. & Malek, K. (2015). Plasma biomarkers of pulmonary hypertension identified by Fourier transform infrared spectroscopy and principal component analysis. *Analyst.* doi: 10.1039/c4an01864h

Stasch, J. P., Becker, E. M., Alonso-Alija, C., Apeler, H., Dembowsky, K., Feurer, A., . . . Schramm, M. (2001). NO-independent regulatory site on soluble guanylate cyclase. *Nature*, *410*(6825), 212-215. doi: 10.1038/35065611

Sutendra, G., Dromparis, P., Bonnet, S., Haromy, A., McMurtry, M. S., Bleackley, R. C. & Michelakis, E. D. (2011). Pyruvate dehydrogenase inhibition by the inflammatory cytokine TNFalpha contributes to the pathogenesis of pulmonary arterial hypertension. *J Mol Med (Berl)*, *89*(8), 771-783. doi: 10.1007/s00109-011-0762-2

Swaminathan, A. C., Dusek, A. C. & McMahon, T. J. (2015). Treatment-related Biomarkers in Pulmonary Hypertension. *Am J Respir Cell Mol Biol.* doi: 10.1165/rcmb.2014-0438TR

Tan, W., Madhavan, K., Hunter, K. S., Park, D. & Stenmark, K. R. (2014). Vascular stiffening in pulmonary hypertension: cause or consequence? (2013 Grover Conference series). *Pulm Circ*, *4*(4), 560-580. doi: 10.1086/677370

Thenappan, T., Shah, S. J., Rich, S. & Gomberg-Maitland, M. (2007). A USA-based registry for pulmonary arterial hypertension: 1982-2006. *Eur Respir J*, *30*(6), 1103-1110. doi: 10.1183/09031936.00042107

Thomas, M., Ciuclan, L., Hussey, M. J. & Press, N. J. (2013). Targeting the serotonin pathway for the treatment of pulmonary arterial hypertension. *Pharmacol Ther*, *138*(3), 409-417. doi: 10.1016/j.pharmthera.2013.02.002

Wiedemann, R., Ghofrani, H. A., Weissmann, N., Schermuly, R., Quanz, K., Grimminger, F., . . . Olschewski, H. (2001). Atrial natriuretic peptide in severe primary and nonprimary pulmonary hypertension: response to iloprost inhalation. *J Am Coll Cardiol*, *38*(4), 1130-1136.

Wilkins, M. R., Ali, O., Bradlow, W., Wharton, J., Taegtmeyer, A., Rhodes, C. J., . . . Simvastatin Pulmonary Hypertension Trial Study, G. (2010). Simvastatin as a treatment for pulmonary hypertension trial. *Am J Respir Crit Care Med, 181*(10), 1106-1113. doi: 10.1164/rccm.200911-699OC

Wojciak-Stothard, B., Abdul-Salam, V. B., Lao, K. H., Tsang, H., Irwin, D. C., Lisk, C., . . . Wilkins, M. R. (2014). Aberrant chloride intracellular channel 4 expression contributes to endothelial dysfunction in pulmonary arterial hypertension. *Circulation, 129*(17), 1770-1780. doi: 10.1161/CIRCULATIONAHA.113.006797

Wolf, D., Tseng, N., Seedorf, G., Roe, G., Abman, S. H. & Gien, J. (2014). Endothelin-1 decreases endothelial PPARgamma signaling and impairs angiogenesis after chronic intrauterine pulmonary hypertension. *Am J Physiol Lung Cell Mol Physiol, 306*(4), L361-371. doi: 10.1152/ajplung.00277.2013

Xia, Y., Fu, Z., Hu, J., Huang, C., Paudel, O., Cai, S., . . . Sham, J. S. (2013). TRPV4 channel contributes to serotonin-induced pulmonary vasoconstriction and the enhanced vascular reactivity in chronic hypoxic pulmonary hypertension. *Am J Physiol Cell Physiol, 305*(7), C704-715. doi: 10.1152/ajpcell.00099.2013

Zhao, L., Chen, C. N., Hajji, N., Oliver, E., Cotroneo, E., Wharton, J., . . . Wilkins, M. R. (2012). Histone deacetylation inhibition in pulmonary hypertension: therapeutic potential of valproic acid and suberoylanilide hydroxamic acid. *Circulation, 126*(4), 455-467. doi: 10.1161/CIRCULATIONAHA.112.103176

In: Pulmonary Arterial Hypertension … ISBN: 978-1-63482-594-8
Editor: Victoria Estrada

Chapter II

Methods to Study Cellular Plasticity *in vitro* and Pulmonary Vascular Remodeling *in vivo* in Pulmonary Arterial Hypertension

Harika Sabbineni[1] and Payaningal R. Somanath[1,2,*]

[1]Clinical and Experimental Therapeutics, College of Pharmacy, University of Georgia and Charlie Norwood VA Medical Center, Augusta, GA, US;
[2]Department of Medicine and Vascular Biology Center, Georgia Regents University, Augusta, GA, US

Abstract

Pulmonary arterial hypertension (PAH) is a deadly disease with no reliable treatment options available. Uncertainties in the molecular mechanisms and incomplete knowledge on the sequence of events leading to pulmonary arterial hypertension are the major gridlocks in the development of therapeutics for this fatal disease. Research on pulmonary arterial hypertension suffers the lack of proper cellular and animal

* Corresponding author: Payaningal R. Somanath Ph.D., FAHA, Associate Professor, Clinical and Experimental Therapeutics, College of Pharmacy, University of Georgia, HM1200 – Georgia Regents University, Augusta, GA 30912, Phone: 706-721-4250; Fax: 706-721-3994; E-mail: sshenoy@gru.edu.

models. Aim of this chapter is to provide easy to follow protocols supported with clear descriptions of the working principle for each experiment along with a list of all the materials necessary for the successful execution of the experiments. Whereas experimental methods *in vitro* will deal with protocols involved in characterizing the molecular mechanisms leading to fibroblast, endothelial and vascular smooth muscle differentiation into pathological mesenchymal cells. This chapter will also discuss the animal models and drugs currently being used in various laboratories to study mechanisms leading to pulmonary arterial hypertension in rodent and larger animal models.

Introduction

Pulmonary arterial hypertension (PAH), defined by a resting mean pulmonary artery pressure (mPAP) greater than 25 mm Hg, is a progressive fatal disease which leads to right ventricular failure and eventually premature death.(McLaughlin et al., 2004) PAH is characterized by increased vascular resistance and vaso-obliteration. It is associated with poor prognosis and the mean survival time of 3 years from the time of diagnosis.(Dickinson, Bartelds, Borgdorff, & Berger, 2013) There is no cure for this rare disease while all the available therapeutic options treat the symptoms rather than the root cause of disease. In order to be able to develop effective targeted therapies for the treatment of PAH, a thorough understanding of the pathogenesis of the disease, molecular mechanisms contributing to the vascular remodeling and hence the development of PAH is necessary. Treatment goals of PAH include reduction in pulmonary vascular resistance and mPAP and hence alleviate pressure overload on the right ventricle preventing right ventricular heart failure (RVH). Animal models help the researchers to understand the disease pathology better and aid them in investigating the molecular mechanisms. Recapitulation of a disease in animal model is very important because they provide a platform to understand the pathophysiology of a disease and hence test novel therapeutic agents.(Maarman, Lecour, Butrous, Thienemann, & Sliwa, 2013) However, it is important to note that there is no perfect animal model to study any disease as the anatomy, physiology, life span, pathology, mechanistic development of disease, rate of progression etc. vary from humans to animals. Choice of an animal model also depends on multiple factors and it is essential to choose a right model that depicts the pathophysiology of the disease being studied. There are numerous animal models available to study PAH and it is important to choose the right model that facilitates to carry out the proposed research and accommodates appropriate endpoints to be measured. Undoubtedly, these animal models have contributed to our understanding of the disease. Of the several animal models available, chronic hypoxia model and monocrotaline injury model are most commonly used. (Stenmark, Meyrick, Galie, Mooi, & McMurtry, 2009) The animal models for PAH can be broadly categorized into four groups (Table 1) including: 1) Classic models, 2) Alternative models, 3) Knockout models, and 4) Overexpression models. All of these groups are discussed in detail in the first part of this review while the second part focuses on various *in-vitro* and *in-vivo* methods that are helpful in studying pulmonary arterial hypertension.

Table 1. Drugs/therapies shown to attenuate PAH in animal models

Animal Model	Species	Drugs/therapies shown to attenuate PAH in the model
	Classic models	
Chronic Hypoxia (CHP)	Rats/mice	Cardiac glycoside (Digoxin), Inhibitor of microRNA-17 (A-17), Endothelin receptor antagonist (Bosentan), PDK inhibitor (Dichloroacetate), and targeted gene delivery of BMPR-2
Monocrotaline (MCT)	Rats	Serine elastase inhibitors (M249314 or ZD0892), PDGFR inhibitor (Imatinib), Rho kinase inhibitor (Fasudil), Endothelin receptor antagonists (Bosentan), Serotonin transporter inhibitor (Fluoxetine), phosphodiesterase-5 inhibitor (Sildenafil) and Phosphodiesterase-3/4 inhibitor (Pumafentrine), Statins (Simvastatin, Pravastatin, and Rosuvastatin)
	Alternative models	
CHP + MCT	Rats	Sildenafil and Imatinib
MCT + Pneumonectomy	Rats	3-hydroxy-3-methylglutaryl (HMG)-CoA reductase inhibitor (Simvastatin), Diterpenoid epoxide (Triptolide), Immunosuppressant (rapamycin), naturally occurring steroid hormone, dehydroepiandrosterone (DHEA)
SU-5416 + CHP	Rats/mice	Bradykinin antagonist (B-9430), Caspase inhibitor (Z-Asp-2,6-dichlorobenzoyloxymethylketone), and Protein kinase inhibitor (Sorafenib)
Fawn-hooded rats	Rats	Fasudil, Vasoactive intestinal peptide
Pulmonary artery banding	Rats/mice	Dichloroacetate

Table 1. (Continued)

Animal Model	Species	Drugs/therapies shown to attenuate PAH in the model
Schistosomiasis model	Mice	Anthelmenthic drug (Praziquantel)
Knockout models		
BMPR-2	Mice	Targted gene delivery of BMPR-2
Vasoactive intestinal peptide	Mice	VIP replacement therapy
Endothelin receptor-B	Mice	Endothelin receptor antagonist
Neprilysin (NEP-/-)	Mice	Exogenous NEP
Overexpression models		
Interleukin-6	Mice	IL receptor antagonist(Tocilizumab)
S100A4/Mts-1	Mice	virus γHV-68 infection to study the link between viral infections and PAH

Animal Models of PAH

I. Classic Models

i) Chronic Hypoxia (CHP)

Chronic hypoxia is a commonly observed phenomenon in many diseases such as chronic obstructive pulmonary disease, interstitial lung disease, and sleep apnea, and plays an important role in the development of PAH. (Hislop & Reid, 1976) Normo- and hypobaric hypoxia are used to induce pulmonary arterial hypertension in different animal species including mice, rats, hamsters, dogs and calves. However, rats and mice are the most commonly used animals to induce PAH using hypoxia.

Method: In a classic CHP model, rats/mice are placed either in a ventilated normobaric or hypobaric chamber that maintains hypoxic conditions i.e 10% for 3-4 weeks. The chamber should be maintained at 50% humidity, 5% CO_2 and 22°C during the experiment. The level of oxygen is monitored by a well calibrated autoregulatory control unit, via flushing either nitrogen or room air. Excess humidity in the chamber should be prevented by condensation in a cooling system. CO2 can be continuously removed by soda lime. Cages can be opened at a frequency described in the protocol to clean, supply water and food, and treat the animals as needed. However, frequent opening and closing of the chamber should be avoided to prevent fluctuations in the oxygen levels.(Chovanec et al., 2009; Michelakis et al., 2002; Muramatsu et al., 1997) Rats develop moderate PAH after continuous exposure to hypoxia for atleast 2 weeks, with a doubling of mean pulmonary artery pressure which correlates with the structural changes. They exhibit right ventricular (RV) hypertrophy; however there is little or no evidence of RV failure.

Histological/pathological changes: The CHP model is characterized by pathological vascular remodeling including medial hypertrophy, muscularization of arterioles, eccentric intimal fibrosis of arteries, and also exhibits certain features of vasculopathy. In the alveolar wall, muscularization of small nonmuscular arteries happens quickly and progresses by expressing smooth muscle actin (α-SMA). Following this, the previously muscularized precapillary pulmonary arteries rapidly increase in thickness. Hypertrophy of smooth muscle cells (SMCs) in these vessels is a remarkable feature associated with hypoxia induced vascular remodeling.(Meyrick & Perkett, 1989) The vessel wall also lodges adhesion molecules, cytokines and inflammatory infiltrates.(Frid et al., 2006) Large proximal pulmonary arteries exhibit significant thickening and fibrosis hence resulting in vascular stiffening.(Drexler et al., 2007)

Mechanism: The pathological remodeling could be attributed to one of the many possibilities including differentiation of pericytes, migration of smooth muscle cells, recruitment and differentiation of local fibroblasts, mononuclear cell/progenitor cell recruitment, and transdifferentiation of endothelial cells into mesenchymal-like cells, a phenomenon called endothelial to mesenchymal transition (EndoMT).(R. C. Jones et al., 2008; Stenmark, Fagan, & Frid, 2006) In addition, inflammation appears to play a significant role in the hypoxia-induced remodeling process in at least some strains of rats.

Advantage (s): CHP is a predictable and reproducible model to induce PAH within a specific animal strain.

Limitation(s): CHP in mice/rats does not completely mimic the pulmonary vascular damage seen in humans with PAH and does not cause obstructive intimal lesions in the peripheral pulmonary arteries. CHP model in rodents rarely induces PAH of the same severity as in humans.(Voelkel & Tuder, 2000) There is a lot of variability in the PAH induced by chronic hypoxia between different species of animals. In addition, responses are also greatly affected by age, as younger individuals are more susceptible to the insult.(Stenmark, Fagan, et al., 2006)

Contribution to our understanding: Contribution of the CHP model to our current understanding of the molecular mechanisms involved in the vascular remodeling induced by chronic pulmonary disease and oxygen deprivation is invaluable.(Kantores et al., 2006) It has been recently shown that there is impairment in the signaling pathway that induces vasodilatation irrespective of the expression of inducible nitric oxide synthase.(Xia et al., 2012) This is believed to contribute to CHP-induced PAH and may have major implications for PH associated with chronic obstructive pulmonary disease. Undoubtedly, the rodent model of CHP has provided us with great insights into the vascular remodeling in PAH with respect to the role of growth factors, cytokines, reactive oxygen species, the nitric oxide pathway and involvement of other signaling molecules.(Dahal et al., 2011)

ii) Monocrotaline Injury

Monocrotaline injury model of PAH is characterized by acute/subacute damage of the peripheral vasculature of the lung and other organs. Monocrotaline, a toxic pyrrolizidine alkaloid is extracted from the plant Crotalaria spectabilis and has to be activated *in vivo* by cytochrome-P450 in the liver to form the reactive bifunctional cross-linking compound, monocrotaline pyrrole (MCTP).(Shah, Patel, & Sehgal, 2005) It was first described 40 years ago that repeated oral ingestion of monocrotaline in laboratory rats resulted in the progressive development of PAH due to vascular injury which was later supported by observations from various other animal species.(Kay, Harris, & Heath, 1967). So far, the preferred species for the study of monocrotaline-induced PAH is the rat. Results obtained from mice even when the active metabolite MCTP has been administered were highly variable. Other animal species in which PAH can be studied using MCT include dogs, young beagles etc.(Gust & Schuster, 2001)

Method: In rats PAH can be induced by injection with a single subcutaneous or intraperitoneal injection of 60-80mg/kg of monocrotaline pyrrole (MCTP).(Gomez-Arroyo et al., 2012)

Mechanism: Although till date the mechanism through which monocrotaline induces pulmonary arterial hypertension is not known, it is widely believed that MCT causes direct endothelial damage which is the initial insult that then triggers a series of pathological events resulting in development of severe and eventually lethal PAH.(Jasmin, Lucas, Cernacek, & Dupuis, 2001) Few groups suggested that an early, dramatic accumulation of mononuclear inflammatory cells in the adventia of the small intraacinar vessels increases the pulmonary artery pressure and hence results in vascular remodeling.(Wilson, Segall, Pan, & Dunston, 1989) There is an evidence that it occurs not only in pulmonary arteries but also in veins and precedes smooth muscle hypertrophy in the media. Thus adventitial inflammation, particularly the accumulation of macrophages has more important effects on the pathogenesis of PAH.(Stenmark, Davie, Frid, Gerasimovskaya, & Das, 2006)

Advantage(s): Induction of PAH via MCT models, particularly in rats, can be achieved by a single subcutaneous or intraperitoneal injection of MCTP, thus making it a simple and appealing animal model. It is inexpensive, reproducible and does not require meticulous technical skills.(Gomez-Arroyo et al., 2012)

Limitation(s): Since MCT should be metabolized into its active compound MCTP by cytochrome P-450, and due to the differences in the hepatic metabolism among various species and animals within the same species, the response to monocrotaline is variable. Most treatments for PAH under investigation improve, reverse and prevent the vascular damage caused by MCT and hence PAH, questioning the efficacy of MCT as a reliable animal model.(Gomez-Arroyo et al., 2012) Vasoconstriction is an important mechanism in the experimental MCT model, whereas this is found only in a subset of patients with PAH and hence is evident that the MCT model does not truly depict the pathology observed in humans.

Contribution to our understanding: This is the first experimental animal model that helped us understand the pathophysiology of pulmonary vascular remodeling process. This was explored by studies that investigated the role of genetic mutation in genes responsible for the regulation of apoptosis and proliferation of endothelial and pulmonary artery smooth muscle cells (PASMCs).

II. Alternative Models

i) Monocrotaline and Pneumonectomy

When pulmonary arterial pressure was raised to systemic levels, the effects of monocrotaline on the pulmonary vasculature were enhanced. Monocrotaline administration produced neointimal changes in the large elastic pulmonary arteries in animals in which pulmonary artery anastomosis was created to change the hemodynamics.(Tanaka, Schuster, Davis, Patterson, & Botney, 1996) It was evident that elevated pressure was not sufficient to induce vascular remodeling but also needed an additional insult thus leading to the development of a dual hit animal model, monocrotaline and pneumonectomy to induce PAH.

Method: In this model, left pneumonectomy (surgical removal of a lung) is performed under aseptic conditions and MCTP 60-80 mg/kg is administered via subcutaneous/intraperitoneal route either before or after the pneumonectomy.(Okada et al., 1997) In combination, MCTP induced injury and the changes in blood flow caused by pneumonectomy induced remarkable intimal remodeling in the distal pulmonary arteries.

Mechanism: Okada et al. suggested that shear stress but not stretch or distention was responsible for the neointimal formation in the presence of MCTP injury. Studies by several groups demonstrated that increased pulmonary artery blood flow after pneumonectomy in absence of injury results in only minimal elevation in pulmonary arterial pressure, which is very much similar to what happens in humans. Although extensive studies have not been pursued to explore the mechanisms of this model, it is clear that inflammation and impaired BMPR signaling may be important in the pathogenesis of vascular remodeling.(Nishimura et al., 2003) This is a model of neointimal pulmonary vascular disease.

Histological characteristics: This model exhibits neointimal pulmonary vascular occlusive lesions, consisting of proliferating endothelial and smooth muscle like cells which is characteristic of severe PAH.(Moreno-Vinasco et al., 2008; Nishimura et al., 2003) In addition, this model also shows histological evidence of inflammation.

Limitation(s): This rat model of PAH and human PAH differ in many ways of which the most notable are the rate of disease progression, absence of plexiform lesions in rats, and the absence of genetic mutations. This model has not been thoroughly studied to evaluate the problems associated with monocrotaline rat model including involvement of veins and effects of MCTP on heart and liver. Also, the mechanism of neointimal lesion formation remains unclear.

ii) Chronic hypoxia and Monocrotaline (CHP+MCT)

In an attempt to improve chronic hypoxia induced PAH model and be able to achieve histological features similar to human PAH, chronic hypoxia and monocrotaline model was developed by Morimatsu et al.

Method: Rats are injected intraperitoneally with MCT (60 mg/kg) once in every 20 days for three times and then exposed to hypobaric hypoxia at 380 mmHg, 10%O_2 for 3 weeks in a ventilated hypoxia chamber.(Morimatsu et al., 2012) This improvised model successfully displays severe PAH with characteristic histological features.

Histological Characteristics: In this multiple hit model of PAH, rats develop PAH and RVH with prominent concentric neointimal thickening and abnormal endothelial cell proliferation. They also exhibit plexiform lesions and vascular occlusion caused by fibrin thrombi.(Morimatsu et al., 2012) Interestingly, these histological features are very similar to those seen in the lungs of patients with PAH.

Limitation(s): The reproducibility across animal strains is inconsistent.(Hales, Kradin, Brandstetter, & Zhu, 1983)

iii) Chronic Hypoxia and SU-5416 (CHP+SU-5416)

Mice exposed to CHP exhibit elevated mean pulmonary arterial pressure (mPAP) but do not develop characteristic pulmonary vascular remodeling, compared to rats limiting the use of wild type mouse models.(Hoshikawa et al., 2003) To overcome this limitation, a mouse model of severe PAH was developed by combining CHP and an inhibitor of the vascular endothelial growth factor (VEGF) receptor-2, SU-5416.(Sakao & Tatsumi, 2011) SU-5416 (Sugen) inhibits VEGFR-2, which is important for the survival of endothelial cells and hence causes endothelial apoptosis leading to the development of PAH. Similarly, Taraseviciene-Stewart and co. developed CHP-SU-5416 model of severe PAH in rats to address the etiologic mechanisms involved in the endothelial cell hyperproliferation better.(Taraseviciene-Stewart et al., 2001)

Method: In this mouse model of severe PAH, the mice are injected intraperitoneally once a week with SU-5416 (20 mg/kg) and are exposed to CHP, 10% FiO2 for 3 weeks.(Ciuclan et al., 2011) The protocol for rats is slightly different in which, they receive a single i.p injection of SU-5416 (20 mg/kg) and are then exposed to CHP, 10% FiO2 for 3 weeks.(Ciuclan et al., 2011)

Histological characteristics: CHP+SU-5416 rat model is characterized by pulmonary arterial remodeling resembling plexiform lesions and increased RVH and RV systolic pressure. (Taraseviciene-Stewart et al., 2001) It also exhibits increased vascular SMC proliferation.

Advantage(s): In this model, chronic hypoxia and VEGF receptor blockade together cause severe PAH, which persists and progresses even after the animals are removed from the hypoxia chamber. Unresponsiveness to treatment and irreversibility of pathological features are the two important features that co-relate this model more closely to human PH.

Limitations: There are 4 genes that exhibit altered expression in human hypertensive lungs and in CHP-SU-5416 model which suggests that the mechanism of disease progression might be different. This model does not exhibit perivascular infiltration of monocytes/macrophages which is quite surprising as chronic hypoxia alone causes early and persistent influx of mononuclear cells into the pulmonary arterial wall.

Contribution to our understanding: This fairly new CHP model facilitates the study of angioproliferative features of PAH, apart from the hemodynamic changes.

iv) Fawn- Hooded Rat Model

The fawn-hooded (FH) rat is an outbred strain which is sensitive to hypoxia, developing mild PAH at sea level and severe PH when exposed to mild hypoxia.(Stenmark et al., 2009) FH rats develop PAH within 4 weeks after birth at Denver altitude, and at half this altitude it takes approximately 20–40 weeks of life for them to develop PAH.(Bonnet et al., 2006) FH rat model elucidates certain aspects of the development of PAH with regard to increased PASMC proliferation, resistance to apoptosis, and a switch to glycolytic metabolism similar to that of cancer cells. It has been known that FH rats have (1) immaturely developed lungs with a reduced number of alveoli, (2) an inherited platelet disorder characterized by defective serotonin uptake into platelets, and (3) a chromosome-1 abnormality that disrupts the mitochondrial reactive oxygen species–hypoxia inducible factor alpha (HIF-1α)–potassium channel pathway causing progressive development of PAH.(Stenmark et al., 2009) Other possible mechanisms include superoxide dismutase-2 (SOD-2) downregulation and activation of HIF-1α and pyruvate dehydrogenase kinase (PDK).(Rehman & Archer, 2010) It is interesting to note that FH rats represent the most severe spectrum of hypoxia induced PH in rodents and develop severe PAH and remodeling.(Sato et al., 1992) However, the FH rats also develop systemic hypertension, whereas that does not usually happen in human patients with PAH.

III. Knockout Models

i) BMPR-2 Knockout Model

Mutation in the BMPR-2 gene is most commonly seen in all types of PH, particularly PAH. It was reported that endothelial cells and PASMCs in the lungs of patients with familial or idiopathic PH carry mutations in BMPR-2 gene.(Brock et al., 2014) From the development of PAH in BMPR-2-deficient mice it is evident that BMPR- 2 plays a very important role in the development of PAH.(Beppu et al., 2004)

Model: In this mouse model the BMPR-2 mutant allele of the BMPR-2 gene lacks exons 4 and 5 which encode the transmembrane domain and a portion of the kinase domain of BMPR-2. Heterozygous mice (BMPR-2+/−) survive and reproduce normally, but in PASMCs isolated from these mice, the messenger RNA levels of BMPR-2 are reduced by 50%. This translates to a reduced activation of the signaling molecules smad 1, 5, and 8 in response to BMP-2.

Histological characteristics: Under normal conditions, BMPR-2+/− mice exhibit mild PAH characterized by muscularization and thickening of the pulmonary arteries. When exposed to chronic hypoxia, 11% FiO2 for 3 weeks, they develop vasoconstriction, muscularization of the small pulmonary arteries, and exhibit increased mPAP.(Beppu et al., 2004)

Limitation(s): Major limitations of this model include absence of RVH and the mildness of the PAH severity.(Yasuda, Tada, Tanabe, Tatsumi, & West, 2011) To address these shortcomings, the mice have been genetically modified to express a dominant negative allele for the BMPR-2 gene in PASMCs and these mice undergo vascular remodeling resembling the plexiform lesion as well as develop remarkable PH and RVH.(Yasuda et al., 2011)

ii) Vasoactive Intestinal Peptide Knockout Model

Vasoactive intestinal peptide (VIP) causes pulmonary smooth-muscle relaxation and either neutralizes or attenuates the actions of vasoconstrictors such as endothelin hence exerts vasodilatory effects. VIP is downregulated in the lungs of patients with PAH.(Said et al., 2007)

Model: VIP−/− mice spontaneously develop moderate to severe PAH characterized by pulmonary vascular remodeling, increased muscularization and thickening of the pulmonary arteries, and also exhibits right ventricular heart failure (RVH).

Mechanism: A thorough investigation of the molecular mechanisms contributing to the development of PAH in VIP−/− mice showed that VIP deletion alters gene expression including (1) underexpression of vasodilator and antiproliferative genes, (2) overexpression of vasoconstrictor and pulmonary vascular remodeling genes, and (3) upregulation of inflammatory genes.(Hamidi, Prabhakar, & Said, 2008) In addition, VIP is implicated in an anti-inflammatory role due to suppression of tumor necrosis factor-alpha and interleukin-10 and upregulation of T-regulatory cells.(Szema, Hamidi, Koller, & Martin, 2011)

Limitation(s): VIP−/− model of PAH differs from human PAH in terms of hemodynamic severity and histological features.(Said et al., 2007)

Contribution to our understanding: The VIP knockout model has not only provided us with great insights into development of PAH but also supports exogenous VIP therapy as treatment strategy for PAH.(Said & Hamidi, 2011) VIP replacement therapy (500 μg/kg/daily, intraperitoneally for 3 weeks) has proven efficacious in reversing PAH and correcting gene alterations in the VIP−/− mice. Knowledge gained from this approach has formed a valuable basis for a possible treatment option for patients with PAH.

iii) Endothelin Receptor-B Knockout Model

Endothelin (ET) is a peptide with potent vasoactive properties and the ability to regulate vascular tone in the normal lung. The actions of ET are receptor dependent with receptors A (ETA) and B (ETB). ETA is localized mainly in PASMCs whose activation leads to PASMC proliferation and vasoconstriction. However, ETB is expressed in both endothelial cells and PASMCs. Activation of the endothelial ETB causes vasodilatation via the release of nitric oxide and prostaglandin while stimulation of theETB on PASMC causes vasoconstriction in the lungs.(Ivy et al., 2001) In 2001, transgenic rats with a deficiency in endothelin-B (ETB) receptor were created that develop severe PAH with increased mPAP and pulmonary vascular resistance and diminished cardiac output after exposure to hypobaric hypoxia.(Senzaki et al., 2002) Together, these data show that reduced expression of endothelin receptors increases pulmonary endothelin levels and thereby contributes to development of PAH.

iv) Neprilysin Knockout Model

Neprilysin or neural endopeptidase (NEP), a transmembrane metallopeptidase is widely expressed in the lung, heart, and peripheral blood vessels. In vasculature, NEP is expressed in PASMCs, fibroblasts, and endothelial cells, and is associated with growth and contraction. In lungs of PAH patients, there is an approximately 70% reduction in the NEP activity.

Model: In 2009, Dempsey et al. created neprilysin null (NEP−/−) mice and exposed them to either normoxia or hypoxia for 5 weeks.(Dempsey et al., 2009)

Histological characteristics: NEP−/− mice develop severe PH characterized by muscularization of the distal pulmonary arteries, thickening of the proximal media, and adventitia with RVH.

Also, it was shown that a striking increase in PASMC proliferation was corrected when isolated PASMCs were treated with exogenous NEP. Together, these results highlight the significance of NEP in the pulmonary vasculature and its role in the pathogenesis of PAH, although not yet been fully elucidated.(Carpenter & Stenmark, 2001)

Overexpression Models

i) Interleukin-6 Overexpression Model

Interleukin-6 (IL-6) is a proinflammatory cytokine, produced mainly by T cells and macrophages. Smooth muscle cells of the tunica media in the vascular wall and adventitia also produce IL-6 to some extent. (Steiner et al., 2009)

Model: In 2009, transgenic mice overexpressing lung-specific interleukin-6 (IL-6) were created by Steiner and colleagues. Investigators exposed IL-6-overexpressing mice to CHP of 10% FiO2 for 3 weeks at sea level.

Histological characteristics: These mice exhibit elevated RV systolic pressure and RVH with pulmonary vasculopathic changes. Additionally, thet develop muscularization of the proximal arterial tree, with proliferative arteriopathy like that seen in the distal arteriolar vessels of patients with PAH.

Mechanism: In PAH, IL-6 promotes the development and progression of pulmonary vascular remodeling by activating signaling pathways that increase endothelial cell proliferation and the expression of anti-apoptotic proteins.

ii) S100A4/Mts-1 Overexpression Model

S100A4/ Mts-1 is a metastasis-promoting protein that forms part of a family of calcium-binding proteins. It is associated with cell proliferation, differentiation, cytoskeleton dynamics, and apoptosis.

Model: In 1998, Ambartsumian and colleagues created transgenic mice that overexpress S100A4/Mts-1. In these mice, the S100A4 coding sequences were placed in such a way that they are driven by mouse mammary tumor virus long terminal repeat promoter (MMTV LTR).(Ambartsumian et al., 1998) S100A4/Mts-1 gene expression was higher in the lungs of females, compared to those of males, and this was translated as a greater Mts-1 protein expression in distal pulmonary arteries. Since PAH is a major complication of HIV, and in addition, the involvement of a latent infection with the human herpes virus-8 (Kaposi's sarcoma–associated herpes virus) has been highly prevalent in patients with idiopathic PAH. (Merklinger et al., 2005). In order to improvise the model and establish a link between viral infection and the development of PH, viral components were introduced into the model. Spiekerkoetter et al. infected 1-year-old S100A4/Mts1-overexpressing mice with the vasculotrophic virus γHV-68 (murine gammaherpesvirus-68). Six months later, the investigators observed perivascular inflammation and occlusive neointimal formation, which was accompanied by significant degradation of elastin.

Histological characteristics: Female mice develop plexiform lesions and develop increased RV systolic pressure while males remain unaffected.

Mechanism: Access of virus to the vessel wall may be a key determinant of the severity of vascular pathology following viral reactivation.

Advantage(s): A reason for using this model to study PAH is that it produces vascular changes like neointimal thickening and plexiform lesions which are characteristic of severe PAH.

Contribution to our understanding: When human primary PASMCs isolated from patients with PAH were treated with physiological concentrations of 17β-estradiol, there was an increase in S100A4/Mts-1 expression. Together, the histological and physiological findings provide a possible explanation for the gender differences which are prominent in human idiopathic PAH.(Dempsie et al., 2011)

Methods to Study PAH

In-vitro Methods

I. Isolation and Culture of Primary Cells

i) Human pulmonary artery endothelial cells from transplant donors

This method describes the protocol for isolation of endothelial cells from human pulmonary artery from donors undergoing heart transplantation. (Visner et al., 1994)

1. Place the segments of human pulmonary artery obtained from donors in lactated Ringer solution or normal saline.
2. Rinse the specimens with sterile phosphate-buffered saline (PBS), pH 7.5, followed by removal of excess tissue from the artery.
3. Place the artery in l0-15 ml PBS containing 1 mg/ml type 1 collagenase (295 units/mg; Sigma) and keep at 37°C for 15 min.
4. Cut the artery lengthwise, laid flat, and scrape the intimal surface gently with a no. 10 scalpel blade.
5. Place the scraped cells in medium 199 containing 10% fetal bovine serum (FBS) (ICN) and antibiotics (ABAM, Sigma) and collect by centrifugation at 800 g for 10 min at 4°C.
6. Resuspend the cell pellet in medium 199 containing 20% FBS, 2 mM glutamine, insulin, transferrin, and sodium selenite media supplement (Sigma; 5 kg/ml insulin, 5 pg/ml human transferrin, and 5 ng/ml sodium selenite), 15 units/ml heparin (Sigma), bovine retinal-derived growth factor (1 vial/200 ml media; ENDO-RET GF, Endotech), and then plate onto a 0.02% gelatin coated T25 flask.
7. Incubate the cells overnight at 37°C in room air-5% CO2 and change media at 24 h and every 2 days until cells become confluent.
8. Remove the cells from the flask with 0.25% trypsin and 0.02 mM EDTA and pass at a ratio of 1:2 or 1:3.
9. Identify cell monolayers as endothelial cells by phase-contrast and transmission electron microscopy (EM).

ii) Isolation of pulmonary artery smooth muscle cells

Isolated primary pulmonary artery smooth muscle cells can be cultured and treated with various drugs to evaluate their efficacy or cytokines to perform functional assays.

Protocol adopted from (Yang et al., 2012)

Method

1. Isolate intralobar PAs (300–800 µm) and remove the endothelium by gently rubbing the luminal surface with a cotton swab.
2. Allow the deendothelialized PAs to recover for 30 min in cold (4°C) HBSS, followed by 20 min in reduced-Ca^{2+} (20 µM) HBSS at room temperature.
3. Digest the tissue at 37°C for 20 min in 20 µM Ca^{2+} HBSS containing collagenase (type I; 1,750 U/ml), papain (9.5 U/ml), BSA (2 mg/ml), and dithiothreitol (1 mM) and then wash with Ca^{2+}-free HBSS to stop digestion.
4. Disperse PASMCs gently by trituration with a small-bore pipette in Ca^{2+}-free HBSS at room temperature. Place the cells on 25-mm glass coverslips.

Histological and Morphological Analysis

1. Hematoxylin and Eosin (H&E) Staining

has been widely used for a very long time to identify various tissue types and changes in the morphology. Hematoxylin has a deep blue-purple color and stains nucleic acids while eosin is pink and stains proteins. In a typical tissue, nuclei are stained blue, whereas the cytoplasm and extracellular matrix have varying degrees of pink staining. H&E staining is one of the most commonly employed techniques to study histological and morphological changes in pulmonary artery in experimental PAH animals and is also used for diagnostic purposes.(Fischer, Jacobson, Rose, & Zeller, 2008)

H&E Staining of Frozen Sections of Pulmonary Artery

Method

1. Air dry the frozen sections for several minutes to remove moisture.
2. Stain with filtered 0.1% Mayers Hematoxylin (Sigma) for 10 minutes in a 50 ml conical tube.
3. In a Coplin jar, rinse the slide in cool running ddH2O for 5 minutes.
4. Dip the slide in 0.5% Eosin (1.5g dissolved in 300ml of 95% EtOH) 12 times.
5. Dip the slide in distilled H2O until the eosin stops streaking But Don't overwash.
6. Dip the slide in 50% EtOH 10 times
7. Dip the slide in 70% EtOH 10 times
8. Equilibrate in 95% EtOH for 30 seconds.
9. Equilibrate in 100% EtOH for 1 minute.
10. Dip the slide in Xylene several times.
11. Clean the slide with a kimwipe; mount and coverslip with Cytoseal XYL (Stephens Scientific)

H&E Staining for Parrafin Sections of Pulmonary Artery

Method

1. Melt paraffin off slides @ 65° C for 20 minutes.
2. Treat with Xylene twice for 10 minutes each.
3. Treat with 100% EtOH twice for 5 minutes each.
4. Air dry slides and stain with filtered 0.1% Mayers Hematoxylin for 10 minutes in a Coplin jar.
5. Rinse the slide in cool running ddH2O for 5 minutes
6. Stain with Eosin (0.5% in 95%EtOH) 12 times.
7. Dip the slide in distilled H2O until the eosin stops streaking.—Do not overwash.
8. Dip the slide in 50% EtOH 10 times
9. Dip the slide in 70% EtOH 10 times
10. Equilibrate in 95% EtOH for 30 seconds.
11. Equilibrate in 100% EtOH for 1 minute.

12. Dip the slide in Xylene several times.
13. Clean slide with a kimwipe; mount and coverslip with Cytoseal XYL

2. Masson's Trichrome Staining

As the name indicates there are three different colors in this stain which stain as follows- collagen stains in blue, nuclei stain in black, and muscle, cytoplasm and keratin stain in red. It is mostly used to differentiate between collagen and smooth muscle in tumors, and the increase of collagen in various extracellular matrix diseases. Sections of pulmonary artery, lungs and heart of PAH animal can be examined for collagen deposition to identify vascular remodeling changes.(Wang, Chen, Li, Ma, & Tang, 2015)

Method

Solutions and Reagents:

1. Bouin's Solution:
    - Picric acid (saturated)-75 ml
    - Formaldehyde (37-40%)-25 ml
    - Glacial acetic acid-5 ml

    Mix well. This solution will improve the quality of Masson Trichrome staining.
2. Weigert's Iron Hematoxylin Solution:

    Stock Solution A:
    - Hematoxylin - 1 g
    - 95% Alcohol -100 ml

    Stock Solution B:
    - 29% Ferric chloride in water - 4 ml
    - Distilled water - 95 ml
    - Hydrochloric acid, concentrated -1ml

    Weigert's Iron Hematoxylin Working Solution:

    Mix equal parts of stock solution A and B. If stored properly, this working solution is stable for 3 months

    Biebrich Scarlet-Acid Fuchsin Solution:
    - Biebrich scarlet, 1% aqueous - 90 ml
    - Acid fuchsin, 1% aqueous -10 ml
    - Acetic acid, glacial -1 ml

Phosphomolybdic-Phosphotungstic Acid Solution:

- 5% Phosphomolybdic acid - 25 ml
- 5% Phosphotungstic acid - 25 ml

Aniline Blue Solution:

- Aniline blue - 2.5 g
- Acetic acide, glacial - 2 ml
- Distilled water - 100 ml

1% Acetic Acid Solution:

- Acetic acid, glacial -1 ml
- Distilled water - 99 ml

Procedure

1. Deparaffinize and rehydrate through 100% alcohol, 95% alcohol 70% alcohol.
2. Wash in distilled water.
3. For Formalin fixed tissue, re-fix in Bouin's solution for 1 hour at 56 C to improve staining quality although this step is not absolutely necessary.
4. Rinse running tap water for 5-10 minutes to remove the yellow color.
5. Stain in Weigert's iron hematoxylin working solution for 10 minutes.
6. Rinse in running warm tap water for 10 minutes.
7. Wash in distilled water.
8. Stain in Biebrich scarlet-acid fuchsin solution for 10-15 minutes. Solution can be saved for future use.
9. Wash in distilled water.
10. Differentiate in phosphomolybdic-phosphotungstic acid solution for 10-15 minutes or until collagen is not red.
11. Transfer sections directly (without rinse) to aniline blue solution and stain for 5-10 minutes. Rinse briefly in distilled water and differentiate in 1% acetic acid solution for 2-5 minutes.
12. Wash in distilled water.
13. Dehydrate very quickly through 95% ethyl alcohol, absolute ethyl alcohol (these step will wipe off Biebrich scarlet-acid fuchsin staining) and clear in xylene.
14. Mount with resinous mounting medium.

Hemodynamic Study

1. Measurement of Right Ventricular Systolic Pressure (RVSP) and Right Ventricular Hypertrophy (RVH)

Right heart catheterization:

1. Make an incision in the right side of the animal's neck, and perform dissection to expose the right jugular vein.
2. Insert a catheter into the vein and advanced into the right ventricle.
3. Take a 0.04/0.023-in (OD by ID)-sized polyvinylchloride tubing with a curved tip, filled with heparinized saline and connect the tubing to a Grass pressure transducer and linked to a Grass model 79 polygraph. Record RV systolic pressure (RVSP).
4. This pressure is assumed to be equal to the pulmonary artery pressure in the presence of a normal pulmonary valve.
5. Dissect the right ventricular free wall from the left ventricular septum and weigh the both parts separately on an analytical scale.
6. RVH is assessed by the ratio of weight of right ventricle to that left ventricle plus septum, RVH=RV/(LV+S) (J. E. Jones et al., 2002; Zhang et al., 2014)

2. Intravital Videography

This technique can be used to visualize the subepicardial arterial microvessels in the RV using an intravital needle-probe videomicroscope.

1. A videomicroscope system (VMS-70A; Nihon Kohden) consists of a needle probe, a camera body containing a charge-coupled device camera, a lens with a light guide, a camera controller, a light source, a monitor, and a digital videocassette recorder.
2. The images on the charge-coupled device are converted into color video signals at 30 frames/s and recorded onto digital videotape.
3. To stabilize the visual field for observation of the subepicardial microvessels while the RV was beating, support the rat's heart with a strip of soft elastic bandage, anchored at its four edges, to maintain a constant in situ position.

4. The supporting bandage also acted as a pressure absorber to minimize compression by the probe.
5. Place the tip of the probe gently placed on the surface of the free wall of the RV where it has minimal hemodynamic effects and take images.

Conclusion

The complex pathology and heterogeneity make PAH a difficult disease to treat. During the past decade, a lot has been studied in terms of vascular remodeling and its contribution to the development of PAH. However, there is still a controversy as to what are the major players that trigger this pathology and the underlying molecular mechanisms. This uncertainty translates to animal models as well making it difficult to choose an appropriate animal model that accommodates all aspects of disease pathology. The validity of animal models has been a controversial topic among basic and clinical scientists because of our limited understanding of PAH pathology and its progression. Any animal model will be effective only when it depicts the human disease and allows researchers to develop a clinically relevant treatment strategy. Animal models are invaluable assets to study disease progression, evaluate the efficacy of therapeutic agents and design new treatment strategies. However, the data from these studies cannot be substituted for clinical research because of the inability of animal models to depict the human PAH disease, hemodynamics and histological severity. Hence, with a hope to develop new treatment modalities for PAH, it is important to validate new animal models that closely recapitulate the human disease and pathology and progress the PAH research towards new horizons.

References

Ambartsumian, N., Klingelhofer, J., Grigorian, M., Karlstrom, O., Sidenius, N., Georgiev, G. & Lukanidin, E. (1998). Tissue-specific posttranscriptional downregulation of expression of the S100A4(mts1) gene in transgenic animals. *Invasion Metastasis*, *18*(2), 96-104. doi: 24502

Beppu, H., Ichinose, F., Kawai, N., Jones, R. C., Yu, P. B., Zapol, W. M., . . . Bloch, K. D. (2004). BMPR-II heterozygous mice have mild pulmonary hypertension and an impaired pulmonary vascular remodeling response to prolonged hypoxia. *Am J Physiol Lung Cell Mol Physiol, 287*(6), L1241-1247. doi: 10.1152/ajplung.00239.2004

Bonnet, S., Michelakis, E. D., Porter, C. J., Andrade-Navarro, M. A., Thebaud, B., Bonnet, S., . . . Archer, S. L. (2006). An abnormal mitochondrial-hypoxia inducible factor-1alpha-Kv channel pathway disrupts oxygen sensing and triggers pulmonary arterial hypertension in fawn hooded rats: similarities to human pulmonary arterial hypertension. *Circulation, 113*(22), 2630-2641. doi: 10.1161/CIRCULATIONAHA.105.609008

Brock, M., Samillan, V. J., Trenkmann, M., Schwarzwald, C., Ulrich, S., Gay, R. E., . . . Huber, L. C. (2014). AntagomiR directed against miR-20a restores functional BMPR2 signalling and prevents vascular remodelling in hypoxia-induced pulmonary hypertension. *Eur Heart J, 35*(45), 3203-3211. doi: 10.1093/eurheartj/ehs060

Carpenter, T. C. & Stenmark, K. R. (2001). Hypoxia decreases lung neprilysin expression and increases pulmonary vascular leak. *Am J Physiol Lung Cell Mol Physiol, 281*(4), L941-948.

Chovanec, M., Novotna, J., Wilhelm, J., Hampl, V., Vizek, M. & Herget, J. (2009). Hypercapnia attenuates hypoxic pulmonary hypertension by inhibiting lung radical injury. *Physiol Res, 58 Suppl 2*, S79-85.

Ciuclan, L., Bonneau, O., Hussey, M., Duggan, N., Holmes, A. M., Good, R., . . . Thomas, M. (2011). A novel murine model of severe pulmonary arterial hypertension. *Am J Respir Crit Care Med, 184*(10), 1171-1182. doi: 10.1164/rccm.201103-0412OC

Dahal, B. K., Heuchel, R., Pullamsetti, S. S., Wilhelm, J., Ghofrani, H. A., Weissmann, N., . . . Schermuly, R. T. (2011). Hypoxic pulmonary hypertension in mice with constitutively active platelet-derived growth factor receptor-beta. *Pulm Circ, 1*(2), 259-268. doi: 10.4103/2045-8932.83448

Dempsey, E. C., Wick, M. J., Karoor, V., Barr, E. J., Tallman, D. W., Wehling, C. A., . . . Miller, Y. E. (2009). Neprilysin null mice develop exaggerated pulmonary vascular remodeling in response to chronic hypoxia. *Am J Pathol, 174*(3), 782-796. doi: 10.2353/ajpath.2009.080345

Dempsie, Y., Nilsen, M., White, K., Mair, K. M., Loughlin, L., Ambartsumian, N., . . . Maclean, M. R. (2011). Development of pulmonary arterial hypertension in mice over-expressing S100A4/Mts1 is specific to females. *Respir Res, 12*, 159. doi: 10.1186/1465-9921-12-159

Dickinson, M. G., Bartelds, B., Borgdorff, M. A. & Berger, R. M. (2013). The role of disturbed blood flow in the development of pulmonary arterial hypertension: lessons from preclinical animal models. *Am J Physiol Lung Cell Mol Physiol*, *305*(1), L1-14. doi: 10.1152/ajplung.00031.2013

Drexler, E. S., Quinn, T. P., Slifka, A. J., McCowan, C. N., Bischoff, J. E., Wright, J. E., . . . Shandas, R. (2007). Comparison of mechanical behavior among the extrapulmonary arteries from rats. *J Biomech*, *40*(4), 812-819. doi: 10.1016/j.jbiomech.2006.03.010

Fischer, A. H., Jacobson, K. A., Rose, J. & Zeller, R. (2008). Hematoxylin and eosin staining of tissue and cell sections. *CSH Protoc*, *2008*, pdb prot4986. doi: 10.1101/pdb.prot4986

Frid, M. G., Brunetti, J. A., Burke, D. L., Carpenter, T. C., Davie, N. J., Reeves, J. T., . . . Stenmark, K. R. (2006). Hypoxia-induced pulmonary vascular remodeling requires recruitment of circulating mesenchymal precursors of a monocyte/macrophage lineage. *Am J Pathol*, *168*(2), 659-669. doi: 10.2353/ajpath.2006.050599

Gomez-Arroyo, J. G., Farkas, L., Alhussaini, A. A., Farkas, D., Kraskauskas, D., Voelkel, N. F. & Bogaard, H. J. (2012). The monocrotaline model of pulmonary hypertension in perspective. *Am J Physiol Lung Cell Mol Physiol*, *302*(4), L363-369. doi: 10.1152/ajplung.00212.2011

Gust, R. & Schuster, D. P. (2001). Vascular remodeling in experimentally induced subacute canine pulmonary hypertension. *Exp Lung Res*, *27*(1), 1-12.

Hales, C. A., Kradin, R. L., Brandstetter, R. D. & Zhu, Y. J. (1983). Impairment of hypoxic pulmonary artery remodeling by heparin in mice. *Am Rev Respir Dis*, *128*(4), 747-751.

Hamidi, S. A., Prabhakar, S. & Said, S. I. (2008). Enhancement of pulmonary vascular remodelling and inflammatory genes with VIP gene deletion. *Eur Respir J*, *31*(1), 135-139. doi: 10.1183/09031936.00105807

Hislop, A. & Reid, L. (1976). New findings in pulmonary arteries of rats with hypoxia-induced pulmonary hypertension. *Br J Exp Pathol*, *57*(5), 542-554.

Hoshikawa, Y., Nana-Sinkam, P., Moore, M. D., Sotto-Santiago, S., Phang, T., Keith, R. L., . . . Geraci, M. W. (2003). Hypoxia induces different genes in the lungs of rats compared with mice. *Physiol Genomics*, *12*(3), 209-219. doi: 10.1152/physiolgenomics.00081.2001

Ivy, D., McMurtry, I. F., Yanagisawa, M., Gariepy, C. E., Le Cras, T. D., Gebb, S. A., . . . Abman, S. H. (2001). Endothelin B receptor deficiency potentiates ET-1 and hypoxic pulmonary vasoconstriction. *Am J Physiol Lung Cell Mol Physiol*, *280*(5), L1040-1048.

Jasmin, J. F., Lucas, M., Cernacek, P. & Dupuis, J. (2001). Effectiveness of a nonselective ET(A/B) and a selective ET(A) antagonist in rats with monocrotaline-induced pulmonary hypertension. *Circulation*, *103*(2), 314-318.

Jones, J. E., Mendes, L., Rudd, M. A., Russo, G., Loscalzo, J. & Zhang, Y. Y. (2002). Serial noninvasive assessment of progressive pulmonary hypertension in a rat model. *Am J Physiol Heart Circ Physiol*, *283*(1), H364-371. doi: 10.1152/ajpheart.00979.2001

Jones, R. C., Capen, D. E., Cohen, K. S., Munn, L. L., Jain, R. K. & Duda, D. G. (2008). A protocol for phenotypic detection and characterization of vascular cells of different origins in a lung neovascularization model in rodents. *Nat Protoc*, *3*(3), 388-397. doi: 10.1038/nprot.2007.537

Kantores, C., McNamara, P. J., Teixeira, L., Engelberts, D., Murthy, P., Kavanagh, B. P. & Jankov, R. P. (2006). Therapeutic hypercapnia prevents chronic hypoxia-induced pulmonary hypertension in the newborn rat. *Am J Physiol Lung Cell Mol Physiol*, *291*(5), L912-922. doi: 10.1152/ajplung.00480.2005

Kay, J. M., Harris, P. & Heath, D. (1967). Pulmonary hypertension produced in rats by ingestion of Crotalaria spectabilis seeds. *Thorax*, *22*(2), 176-179.

Maarman, G., Lecour, S., Butrous, G., Thienemann, F. & Sliwa, K. (2013). A comprehensive review: the evolution of animal models in pulmonary hypertension research; are we there yet? *Pulm Circ*, *3*(4), 739-756. doi: 10.1086/674770

McLaughlin, V. V., Presberg, K. W., Doyle, R. L., Abman, S. H., McCrory, D. C., Fortin, T., . . . American College of Chest, P. (2004). Prognosis of pulmonary arterial hypertension: ACCP evidence-based clinical practice guidelines. *Chest*, *126*(1 Suppl), 78S-92S. doi: 10.1378/chest.126.1_suppl.78S

Merklinger, S. L., Wagner, R. A., Spiekerkoetter, E., Hinek, A., Knutsen, R. H., Kabir, M. G., . . . Rabinovitch, M. (2005). Increased fibulin-5 and elastin in S100A4/Mts1 mice with pulmonary hypertension. *Circ Res*, *97*(6), 596-604. doi: 10.1161/01.RES.0000182425.49768.8a

Meyrick, B. O. & Perkett, E. A. (1989). The sequence of cellular and hemodynamic changes of chronic pulmonary hypertension induced by hypoxia and other stimuli. *Am Rev Respir Dis*, *140*(5), 1486-1489. doi: 10.1164/ajrccm/140.5.1486

Michelakis, E. D., McMurtry, M. S., Wu, X. C., Dyck, J. R., Moudgil, R., Hopkins, T. A., . . . Archer, S. L. (2002). Dichloroacetate, a metabolic modulator, prevents and reverses chronic hypoxic pulmonary hypertension in rats: role of increased expression and activity of voltage-gated potassium channels. *Circulation*, *105*(2), 244-250.

Moreno-Vinasco, L., Gomberg-Maitland, M., Maitland, M. L., Desai, A. A., Singleton, P. A., Sammani, S., . . . Garcia, J. G. (2008). Genomic assessment of a multikinase inhibitor, sorafenib, in a rodent model of pulmonary hypertension. *Physiol Genomics*, *33*(2), 278-291. doi: 10.1152/physiolgenomics.00169.2007

Morimatsu, Y., Sakashita, N., Komohara, Y., Ohnishi, K., Masuda, H., Dahan, D., . . . Marthan, R. (2012). Development and characterization of an animal model of severe pulmonary arterial hypertension. *J Vasc Res*, *49*(1), 33-42. doi: 10.1159/000329594

Muramatsu, M., Tyler, R. C., Gutkowska, J., Klinger, J. R., Hill, N. S., Rodman, D. M. & McMurtry, I. F. (1997). Atrial natriuretic peptide accounts for increased cGMP in hypoxia-induced hypertensive rat lungs. *Am J Physiol*, *272*(6 Pt 1), L1126-1132.

Nishimura, T., Vaszar, L. T., Faul, J. L., Zhao, G., Berry, G. J., Shi, L., . . . Kao, P. N. (2003). Simvastatin rescues rats from fatal pulmonary hypertension by inducing apoptosis of neointimal smooth muscle cells. *Circulation*, *108*(13), 1640-1645. doi: 10.1161/ 01.CIR.0000087592. 47401.37

Okada, K., Tanaka, Y., Bernstein, M., Zhang, W., Patterson, G. A. & Botney, M. D. (1997). Pulmonary hemodynamics modify the rat pulmonary artery response to injury. A neointimal model of pulmonary hypertension. *Am J Pathol*, *151*(4), 1019-1025.

Rehman, J. & Archer, S. L. (2010). A proposed mitochondrial-metabolic mechanism for initiation and maintenance of pulmonary arterial hypertension in fawn-hooded rats: the Warburg model of pulmonary arterial hypertension. *Adv Exp Med Biol*, *661*, 171-185. doi: 10.1007/978-1-60761-500-2_11

Said, S. I. & Hamidi, S. A. (2011). Pharmacogenomics in pulmonary arterial hypertension: Toward a mechanistic, target-based approach to therapy. *Pulm Circ*, *1*(3), 383-388. doi: 10.4103/2045-8932.87306

Said, S. I., Hamidi, S. A., Dickman, K. G., Szema, A. M., Lyubsky, S., Lin, R. Z., . . . Kort, S. (2007). Moderate pulmonary arterial hypertension in male mice lacking the vasoactive intestinal peptide gene. *Circulation*, *115*(10), 1260-1268. doi: 10.1161/CIRCULATIONAHA.106.681718

Sakao, S. & Tatsumi, K. (2011). The effects of antiangiogenic compound SU5416 in a rat model of pulmonary arterial hypertension. *Respiration*, *81*(3), 253-261. doi: 10.1159/000322011

Sato, K., Webb, S., Tucker, A., Rabinovitch, M., O'Brien, R. F., McMurtry, I. F. & Stelzner, T. J. (1992). Factors influencing the idiopathic development of pulmonary hypertension in the fawn hooded rat. *Am Rev Respir Dis*, *145*(4 Pt 1), 793-797. doi: 10.1164/ajrccm/145.4_Pt_1.793

Senzaki, H., Masutani, S., Kobayashi, J., Kobayashi, T., Sasaki, N., Asano, H., . . . Ishizawa, A. (2002). Ventricular afterload and ventricular work in fontan circulation: comparison with normal two-ventricle circulation and single-ventricle circulation with blalock-taussig shunts. *Circulation*, *105*(24), 2885-2892.

Shah, M., Patel, K. & Sehgal, P. B. (2005). Monocrotaline pyrrole-induced endothelial cell megalocytosis involves a Golgi blockade mechanism. *Am J Physiol Cell Physiol*, *288*(4), C850-862. doi: 10.1152/ajpcell.00327.2004

Steiner, M. K., Syrkina, O. L., Kolliputi, N., Mark, E. J., Hales, C. A. & Waxman, A. B. (2009). Interleukin-6 overexpression induces pulmonary hypertension. *Circ Res*, *104*(2), 236-244, 228p following 244. doi: 10.1161/CIRCRESAHA.108.182014

Stenmark, K. R., Davie, N., Frid, M., Gerasimovskaya, E. & Das, M. (2006). Role of the adventitia in pulmonary vascular remodeling. *Physiology (Bethesda)*, *21*, 134-145. doi: 10.1152/physiol.00053.2005

Stenmark, K. R., Fagan, K. A. & Frid, M. G. (2006). Hypoxia-induced pulmonary vascular remodeling: cellular and molecular mechanisms. *Circ Res*, *99*(7), 675-691. doi: 10.1161/01.RES.0000243584.45145.3f

Stenmark, K. R., Meyrick, B., Galie, N., Mooi, W. J. & McMurtry, I. F. (2009). Animal models of pulmonary arterial hypertension: the hope for etiological discovery and pharmacological cure. *Am J Physiol Lung Cell Mol Physiol*, *297*(6), L1013-1032. doi: 10.1152/ajplung.00217.2009

Szema, A. M., Hamidi, S. A., Koller, A. & Martin, D. W. (2011). Vasoactive Intestinal Peptide Knockout (VIP KO) mouse model of sulfite-sensitive asthma: up-regulation of novel lung carbonyl reductase. *BMC Immunol*, *12*, 66. doi: 10.1186/1471-2172-12-66

Tanaka, Y., Schuster, D. P., Davis, E. C., Patterson, G. A. & Botney, M. D. (1996). The role of vascular injury and hemodynamics in rat pulmonary artery remodeling. *J Clin Invest*, *98*(2), 434-442. doi: 10.1172/JCI118809

Taraseviciene-Stewart, L., Kasahara, Y., Alger, L., Hirth, P., Mc Mahon, G., Waltenberger, J., . . . Tuder, R. M. (2001). Inhibition of the VEGF receptor 2 combined with chronic hypoxia causes cell death-dependent pulmonary endothelial cell proliferation and severe pulmonary hypertension. *FASEB J*, *15*(2), 427-438. doi: 10.1096/fj.00-0343com

Visner, G. A., Staples, E. D., Chesrown, S. E., Block, E. R., Zander, D. S. & Nick, H. S. (1994). Isolation and maintenance of human pulmonary artery endothelial cells in culture isolated from transplant donors. *Am J Physiol*, *267*(4 Pt 1), L406-413.

Voelkel, N. F. & Tuder, R. M. (2000). Hypoxia-induced pulmonary vascular remodeling: a model for what human disease? *J Clin Invest*, *106*(6), 733-738. doi: 10.1172/JCI11144

Wang, H., Chen, Z., Li, X. J., Ma, L. & Tang, Y. L. (2015). Anti-inflammatory cytokine TSG-6 inhibits hypertrophic scar formation in a rabbit ear model. *Eur J Pharmacol*, *751C*, 42-49. doi: 10.1016/j.ejphar.2015.01.040

Wilson, D. W., Segall, H. J., Pan, L. C. & Dunston, S. K. (1989). Progressive inflammatory and structural changes in the pulmonary vasculature of monocrotaline-treated rats. *Microvasc Res*, *38*(1), 57-80.

Xia, X. D., Xu, Z. J., Hu, X. G., Wu, C. Y., Dai, Y. R. & Yang, L. (2012). Impaired iNOS-sGC-cGMP signalling contributes to chronic hypoxic and hypercapnic pulmonary hypertension in rat. *Cell Biochem Funct*, *30*(4), 279-285. doi: 10.1002/cbf.2796

Yang, X. R., Lin, A. H., Hughes, J. M., Flavahan, N. A., Cao, Y. N., Liedtke, W. & Sham, J. S. (2012). Upregulation of osmo-mechanosensitive TRPV4 channel facilitates chronic hypoxia-induced myogenic tone and pulmonary hypertension. *Am J Physiol Lung Cell Mol Physiol*, *302*(6), L555-568. doi: 10.1152/ajplung.00005.2011

Yasuda, T., Tada, Y., Tanabe, N., Tatsumi, K. & West, J. (2011). Rho-kinase inhibition alleviates pulmonary hypertension in transgenic mice expressing a dominant-negative type II bone morphogenetic protein receptor gene. *Am J Physiol Lung Cell Mol Physiol*, *301*(5), L667-674. doi: 10.1152/ajplung.00423.2010

Zhang, D., Wang, G., Han, D., Zhang, Y., Xu, J., Lu, J., . . . Li, M. (2014). Activation of PPAR-gamma ameliorates pulmonary arterial hypertension via inducing heme oxygenase-1 and p21(WAF1): an in vivo study in rats. *Life Sci*, *98*(1), 39-43. doi: 10.1016/j.lfs.2013.12.208

In: Pulmonary Arterial Hypertension …
Editor: Victoria Estrada
ISBN: 978-1-63482-594-8

Chapter III

Pharmacological Uses of Nifedipine

***Sampath Kumar Ethiraj*[1], *MD*,**
***Joe V. M. Devasahayam*[*2], *MD*,**
***Gowrishankar Erode Singaravelu*[3], *MBBS MRCP*,**
***Tony Oliver*[4], *MD, MRCP*, *Valentina S. Joseph*[5], *MD*,**
***Mandasmitha Sowmarpet*[1], *MD*, *Aparna N. Kurup*[6], *MD*,**
and Unnikrishnan Pillai*[7], *MD

[1]Consultant in Hospital Medicine, Parkview Hospital, Fort Wayne, IN, US
[2]Fellow in Pulmonary and Critical Care Medicine, University of Missouri, Columbia, MO, US
[3]Specialty Physician, Southwest Acute Hospital, Enniskillen, UK
[4]Acedemic Hospitalist, Sanford Medical Center, University of South Dakota, Sioux Falls, SD, US
[5]Senior Resident in Neurology, University of Toledo, Toledo, OH, US
[6]Senior Resident in Internal Medicine, St Mary's Health Center, St Louis, MO, US
[7]Hon Asst Professor/Staff Nephrologist, Indiana University Health Ball memorial hospital, Muncie, IN, US

[*] Corresponding Author. Email: joe29578@hotmail.com.

Abstract

Nifedipine, a widely prescribed dihydropyridine calcium channel blocker, was originally introduced in 1966 as an anti-anginal drug due to its vasodilatory properties. Subsequently, it was found to have many other properties useful for a variety of indications. Nifedipine – Gastro Intestinal Therapeutic System (GITS) formulation has helped overcoming the main drawback of the drug, which is the sudden drop in blood pressure and reflex tachycardia due to fluctuations in plasma concentrations. Nifedipine has been extensively studied across the world in several robust clinical trials, making available a vast body of information in the literature about its pharmacological properties and therapeutic usage. In addition to its anti-anginal effect, Nifedipine also has an established antihypertensive property. It has been well studied in comparison with a number of drugs belonging to most other major antihypertensive classes, both as solitary and combination therapies. Several trials of Nifedipine studied both general and specific groups of population including the elderly, the diabetics and African Americans. It has been shown to have anti-atherosclerotic, anti-oxidant and vasculo-protectant properties. It reduces the carotid artery intima-media thickness and slows down coronary artery calcification. These are beneficial in the reduction of coronary and cerebrovascular events. Its smooth muscle relaxing function is utilised in the symptomatic treatment of Raynaud's disease. This very function is also utilised in the treatment of ureteric calculi, which could potentially prevent invasive interventions for this condition. Nifedipine is as effective as ACE-inhibitors and angiotensin receptor blockers and could be added as an adjunct to them in protecting renal function in diabetes. It is also comparable to these classes of drugs in reducing left ventricular mass in left ventricular hypertrophy resulting from hypertension. Nifedipine also has utility as a first line tocolytic in prolongation of pregnancy to avoid preterm labor. It is superior to Ritodrine, a beta receptor agonist, in terms of delaying labor, clinically important neonatal outcomes and maternal adverse events.

Introduction

Nifedipine is a dihydropyridine (DHP) calcium channel blocker (CCB) synthesized by Bayer, Germany in 1966 [1]. At the time of its introduction, it was thought to possess coronary vasodilatation properties- at least when given in small doses. It was initially developed as an anti-anginal medication and subsequently used for other clinical conditions which will be discussed below.

Since the introduction of its Gastrointestinal therapeutic system (GITS) formulation, Nifedipine GITS has gained the attention of researchers and in course of time, it has achieved huge clinical significance as an anti-hypertensive, smooth muscle relaxant, anti-atherosclerotic ,anti-inflammatory , antioxidant [2], tocolytic and vasculo- protectant [3]. In this chapter, the therapeutic uses of Nifedipine will be discussed in detail.

Nifedipine GITS (Gastrointestinal Therapeutic System)

Nifedipine initially was developed as an anti-anginal and then utilized for the treatment of hypertension. The immediate release preparations of Nifedipine had problems for clinical use in hypertension since its plasma concentration had fluctuations and lead to abrupt vasodilation and sympathetic nervous system activation that in turn caused unwanted side effects like tachycardia.

In order to prevent this, GITS formulation was developed and introduced. Nifedipine GITS has smooth and uniform drug release using an osmotic pump that releases the drug through a laser drilled hole in an inert shell at a controlled rate. [4] After the introduction of the GITS formulation, Nifedipine has wider usage in clinical practice with lesser adverse effects.

Nifedipine As an Anti-Hypertensive

Mechanism of Action

Nifedipine acts primarily by inhibiting the L type channels in vascular smooth muscles. [5] The hemodynamic effects include vasodilation of larger systemic arteries leading to decrease in the peripheral vascular resistance and decrease in left ventricular afterload, and thereby works as an effective antihypertensive medication. Nifedipine increases arterial wall compliance and thus alters its hemodynamics and in turn reduces the blood pressure. [6]

Efficacy of Nifedipine in Hypertension

Nifedipine's efficacy was compared with other DHPs as well. Comparing Nifedipine GITS 30mg and amlodipine 5mg over 21 weeks, no significant difference in systolic or diastolic blood pressure was demonstrated. Mean decrease in systolic blood pressure (SBP) and diastolic blood pressure (DBP) for Nifedipine were 18.8 mmHg and 15.5 mm Hg respectively as opposed to Amlodipine, which dropped SBP by 19.7 mmHg and DBP by 15.7 mmHg. [7]

Nifedipine GITS 90 mg compared to Propranolol SR 240 mg over a period of 8 weeks showed a drop of 15.9 mmHg in mean systolic blood pressure compared to 5.7 mmHg for the beta blocker ($p<0.001$). The authors concluded that Nifedipine GITS was more efficacious than sustained release Propranolol in reducing sitting systolic and diastolic blood pressures, as well as standing systolic blood pressure. [3] Another study done in 1987 showed that the efficacy of Nifedipine was similar to Hydrochlorthiazide. [8]

Schulte et al compared Nifedipine GITS 30/60 mg with Enalapril 5/10 mg over a period of 8 weeks and showed a drop of systolic blood pressure from 141±15 mmHg to 134±14 mmHg with Nifedipine GITS as opposed to 140±15 mmHg to 131±15 mmHg with Enalapril. This trial showed that Nifedipine GITS and Enalapril were comparably effective anti-hypertensive drugs. [9]

Nifedipine 30-90 mg was compared to Losartan 50 mg with or without Hydrochlorothiazide 12.5/25 mg combination over 12 weeks and it showed comparable reductions in systolic blood pressure between the two study groups. [10]

ADVANCE-combi study concluded that controlled release Nifedipine combined with Valsartan was superior to Amlodipine combined with Valsartan in blood pressure reduction, without any significant difference in the incidence of drug related adverse events. [11]

A large multicentric observation study on Nifedipine GITS 30 to 60 mg daily monotherapy has shown to be effective in achieving target goals in diabetic (<130/80) and non-diabetic (<140/90)(JNC7) and hence ascertained the tolerability and efficacy of long acting Nifedipine in day to day clinical setting. [12]

Nifedipine GITS 30 mg daily was as effective as Co-amiloride (Amiloride with Hydrochlorthiazide-(25/2.5 mg) in hypertensive diabetic population. Serious adverse effects like hyperglycemia and hyperuricemia were less common with Nifedipine GITS, however peripheral edema became a huge problem and only few people could tolerate that. [13]

Antihypertensive Efficacy in Specific Population Groups

Efficacy in Elderly Population

The STONE trial included older age population (60-79 years) in a study over 2.5 years, and compared Nifedipine 10-30 mg bid with placebo found a relative risk reduction of 62% in combined cardiovascular outcomes. [14] Similarly, JMIC-B trial which compared Nifedipine retard 10-20 mg bid with Enalapril or Imidapril 5-10 mg daily, or Lisinopril 10-20 mg daily in patients aged over 75 years found that Nifedipine retard was as effective as angiotensin converting enzyme inhibitors in reducing the incidence of cardiac events and mortality. INSIGHT trials compared Nifedipine 30-60 mg daily with Co-amiloride (25-50/2.5-5 mg) daily in patients aged 55-80 years, and found that Nifedipine was equally effective in preventing overall cardiovascular or cerebrovascular complications. [15]

Antihypertensive Effect of Nifedipine in African American Patients

Hall et al, compared Nifedipine-GITS 30-60 mg OD vs Nifedipine-Coat core (CC) 30-60 mg and Amlodipine 5-10 mgs OD and found that drop in the SBP was 12, 16 and 14 mmHg in SBP at the end of study respectively and DBP drop was 6, 9, and 9 mmHg. [16] Nifedipine-GITS also showed adequate response in blood pressure when used between 30-90 mg daily when compared to a combination of captopril and HCTZ (25-50/ 15-25 mg) daily. [17]

Efficacy of Nifedipine in Hypertension in Diabetic Population

ACE inhibitors and angiotensin receptor blockers are well established in diabetic populations and are usually the first line medications for hypertension due to their role in preventing microalbuminuria. However Nifedipine-GITS 20 mg daily had comparable results with Telmisartan 40 mg OD in reducing the blood pressure, though its effect in microalbuminuria could not be clearly established. [18] Nifedipine Retard compared to Lisinopril once daily over 24 weeks resulted with similar decrease in SBP and thus could be used in these populations as well. [19]

Nifedipine As Anti-anginal/Vasodilator

The medications that are used for coronary artery disease (CAD) ideally should not only reduce the symptoms, but also be able to prevent the serious CAD related untoward events and decrease the progression of the disease. Nifedipine was initially introduced as an anti-anginal medication; its mechanism of action being vasodilation, it was used for the treatment of angina pectoris. Nifedipine dilates the coronary arteries, inhibits coronary artery spasm and increases the blood flow to myocardium. It also decreases myocardial oxygen consumption and reduces the incidence of development of left ventricular hypertrophy (LVH) in chronically hypertensive patients. Nifedipine has beneficial effects on LVH, relatively lesser bradycardia when compared to other drug classes like beta blockers. Longer acting Nifedipine preparations actually have lower activation of sympathetic nervous system.

Also modified release Nifedipine reduced the incidence of angina attacks comparable to beta blockers. Comparing Nifedipine Retard 20 mg bid with Carvedilol 25 mg bid, the number of attacks were 78 and 89 respectively over 4 weeks. Similarly Savonitto et al, compared Nifedipine retard 20 mg bid and Metoprolol –CR 200 mg once daily and the number of angina attacks were 25 and 36 over 6 weeks. [20]

Effect of Nifedipine in Reducing Left Ventricular Mass

The beneficial effect of Nifedipine -GITS in reducing left ventricular (LV) mass in hypertensive patients has been well studied in the PRESERVE trial and showed surprising results. [21] After 48 weeks of treatment, the LV mass index got reduced by 17g/m2 (13%) comparable to Enalapril which reduced LV mass by 15 g/m2 (15%) from the baseline.

Also, after 24 weeks of treatment with Nifedipine retard 20-40 mg bid, the LV mass index achieved 16% reduction from the baseline and was similar to the effect seen by using perindopril 4-8 mg OD which showed 14% change from the baseline and was statistically significant. [22]

Nifedipine As Anti-atherosclerotic and Anti-Inflammatory

Vasculo-protection by Nifedipine is by inhibiting the pro-arteriosclerotic protein (MCP-1) expression in the blood vessel as demonstrated in both animal and cloned human cell models. It also inhibits vascular smooth muscle growth. [4]

Its antioxidant function helps in the restoration of Nitric oxide availability in the endothelium and protects the peripheral arteries both in small and larger arteries. In animal models, it has shown to reduce brain damage after transient ischemic attack and by its antioxidant effects. In experiments with rats, it has been demonstrated to reduce the aortic aneurysm extension by its vasculo-protection action.

Nifedipine As a Vasculo-protectant

A coronary disease trial investigating the outcomes with usage of Nifedipine GITS (ACTION) is one of the largest trials which studied 3825 patients who were more than 35 years of age with CAD and had stable angina pectoris for more than one month. Nifedipine retard was shown to reduce atherosclerotic plaque volume and to improve cholinergic effect in the coronary arteries in the Japanese population and thereby reduced overt heart failure and mortality rate. [23, 24]

Nifedipine showed inhibitory action on Carotid Artery thickening and decreased progression of Intima media thickness (IMT). Common carotid artery IMT progression has been compared between the use of Nifedipine 30 mg and co-amiloride (25/2.5mg) and was showed that IMT thickness progressed significantly on co-amiloride but not on Nifedipine. [25] Also Nifedipine slows coronary artery calcification and hence decreased the relapse rate of cardiovascular events and strokes. [26] Various other studies have used other calcium channel blockers (both DHP and non-DHP) and have shown no beneficial results in reducing carotid IMT and hence prove the peculiar nature of Nifedipine for this use.

Japan multicenter investigation for cardiovascular diseases-B (JMIC-B) has showed that Nifedipine is better than ACE inhibitors in inhibiting the coronary atherosclerotic progression and decreased coronary artery stenosis with angiographic evidence in the Japanese population. [27] Nifedipine restores endothelial functions, reduces incidences of coronary events and slows the atherosclerotic progression.

Nifedipine in Raynaud's Phenomenon

Systemic sclerosis (Scleroderma) involves fibrosis of the GI tract and hence reduces the GI motility causing impairment clearance of food and retention of the food in the GI tract. Raynaud's syndrome has association with systemic sclerosis and is part of the CREST syndrome. Raynaud's syndrome being caused by vasospasm has been effectively treated with calcium channel blockers including Nifedipine. [28] However in general, CCBs are found to cause higher incidence of gastric acid reflux and hence need to be used with caution in these patient groups.

Nifedipine As Reno-protectant in Diabetics

Several studies has focused on the effect on Nifedipine on renal function and the largest among them is INSIGHT (International Nifedipine GITS Study: Intervention as a Goal in Hypertension Treatment) It showed that in high risk hypertensive patients, Nifedipine GITS was compared with Co-amiloride over the course of 3-5 years and was found that the renal function was better preserved with Nifedipine GITS. [9]

The combination of Nifedipine and candesartan for patients with uncontrolled hypertension has been shown to be effective antihypertensive and renal protectant when compared to usage of an angiotensin receptor blocker (ARB) alone. [29]

In Japanese hypertensive population with diabetes mellitus, Nifedipine decreased the micro albuminuria rate after 2 years comparable to ACE inhibitor and can be used as Reno-protectant agent in patients with diabetes and hypertension. [30]

Nifedipine in Obstetrics

Nifedipine is a first line tocolytic agent indicated in the short term prolongation of pregnancy by inhibiting preterm labor and birth. [31] Myometrial contractions are mediated through ATP-dependent binding of myosin to actin. This interaction is dependent upon the phosphorylation of myosin light chain by a calcium/calmodulin dependent enzyme called myosin light chain kinase. Hence, myometrial contractility ultimately depends upon the availability of free intracellular calcium. [32] By directly blocking the influx of calcium ions through the cell membrane, inhibiting the release of intracellular calcium from the sarcoplasmic reticulum and increasing calcium efflux from the cell, Nifedipine causes fall in the intracellular free calcium level, resulting in inhibition of myometrial contraction.

In a 2014 systematic review and meta-analysis of 38 randomised trials (3550 women) of Calcium Channel Blockers; all but three trials used Nifedipine as the CCB drug studied - for treatment of preterm labor, and use of CCBs reduced the risk of delivery within 48 hours of trial entry compared to placebo or no treatment. [33] CCBs showed significant benefits over Ritodrine, a beta-adrenergic-receptor agonist, with respect to prolongation of pregnancy, clinically important neonatal outcomes (respiratory distress syndrome, necrotizing enterocolitis, intraventricular hemorrhage, neonatal jaundice, admission to the Neonatal intensive care unit (NICU), (and length of stay in the NICU) and maternal adverse effects. Nifedipine may also have some benefits over Atosiban, an oxytocin receptor antagonist and Magnesium sulfate.

Possible side effects of Nifedipine in pregnant women include nausea, flushing, headache, dizziness, palpitations and elevation of hepatic transaminases. When used with Magnesium sulfate, it can also cause hypotension, suppression of heart rate, cardiac contractility, and left ventricular systolic pressure. Severe hypotension due to decreased peripheral vascular resistance has been reported. [34] However patients without underlying myocardial dysfunction have compensatory increase in cardiac output which generally maintains blood pressure. By comparison, Ritodrine was more frequently associated with adverse cardiovascular effects. Symptomatic hypocalcemia has also been reported when used with Magnesium sulphate. [35]

Currently, there are no definite data regarding fetal side effects with Nifedipine at the oral doses used for inhibition of preterm labor. Studies using sublingual doses of Nifedipine have not shown any adverse effects in humans [36], despite some adverse effects reported in animal models. Contraindications include known hypersensitivity, hypotension or preload dependent cardiac lesions such as aortic insufficiency. The American College of Obstetricians and Gynaecologists suggests a 30 mg loading dose followed by 10 to 20 mg every 4 to 6 hours if uterine contractions continue. Recommended maximum daily dose is 180 mg. Immediate acting Nifedipine is not recommended in hypertension during pregnancy due to potential adverse effects related to sudden reduction in blood pressure.

Role in the Expulsion of Ureteric Calculi

Nifedipine's role in expulsion of ureteric calculi was studied in various trials, and has been found that Nifedipine given along with prednisone achieved significant reduction in expulsion time when compared to placebo-thus proving its supremacy. Nifedipine possesses the smooth muscle relaxation property and hence increases ureteric peristalsis and in turn expels the calculi quicker. [37]

Nifedipine in High Altitude Pulmonary Edema (HAPE)

Nifedipine decreases the pulmonary artery systolic pressure and pulmonary vascular bed resistance by its smooth muscle relaxation properties and hence it was studied for its role in high altitude pulmonary edema. However interestingly, Nifedipine provided no additional benefit in the resolution of HAPE. [38]

Conclusion

Nifedipine is a dihydropyridine calcium channel blocker that has a predominant vasodilator activity. Nifedipine GITS is well tolerated and is a very effective anti-hypertensive medication because of the gradual onset of action and less sympathetic stimulation, and also reduces the unwanted side effects. Nifedipine modified release formulations are also generally well tolerated and are effective anti-hypertensive and anti-anginal medications. Nifedipine is also particularly effective in African American, elderly and diabetic populations as an effective antihypertensive, anti- anginal, vascular and reno- protectant. Among the patients with vasculopathies, it has been shown to have anti atherosclerotic effects and effective in reducing the carotid artery wall IMT thickness. Nifedipine is well demonstrated as an effective tocolytic and without much benefit in the treatment of high altitude pulmonary edema.

References

[1] Croom KF, Wellington K, Steffen H. A Review of the Use of Modified-Release Formulations in the Treatment of Hypertension and Angina Pectoris. 2006;66(4):497-528.

[2] Horiuchi M. [Anti-inflammatory effect of nifedipine and vasculoprotection]. *Drugs* 2006;66 Spec No(1):28-30.

[3] Frishman WH, Garofalo JL, Rothschild A, et al 1989: Nifedipine GITS in the treatment of hypertension. Am J Cardiol. 64:65F- 9F.

[4] Lundy A, Lutfi N, Beckey C. Review of nifedipine GITS in the treatment of high risk patients with coronary artery disease and hypertension. *Vasc. Health Risk Manag.* 2009;5(1):429-40.

[5] Murdoch D, Brogden RN. Sustained release nifedipine formulations. An appraisal of their current uses and prospective roles in the treatment of hypertension, ischaemic heart disease and peripheral vascular disorders. *Drugs* 1991;41(5):737-79.

[6] Yamagishi S, Nakamura K, Matsui T. Role of oxidative stress in the development of vascular injury and its therapeutic intervention by nifedipine. *Curr. Med. Chem.* 2008;15(2):172-7.

[7] Testa MA, Turner RR, Simonson DC, et al. Quality of life and calcium channel blockade with nifedipine GITS versus amlodipine in hypertensive patients in Spain. Gastrointestinal Therapeutic System. *J. Hypertens.* 1998;16(12 Pt 1):1839-47.

[8] Gavras I, Mulinari R, Gavras H, et al. Antihypertensive effectiveness of the nifedipine gastrointestinal therapeutic system. *Am. J. Med.* 1987;83(6B):20-3.

[9] Schulte KL, Lenz T, Fischer M, et al. Underestimation of 24-hour hypotensive efficacy of nifedipine GITS versus enalapril: ambulatory recording as an adjunct to clinical blood pressure measurement. *Blood Press.* 2000;9(4):221-6.

[10] Weir MR, Elkins M, Liss C, et al. Efficacy, tolerability, and quality of life of losartan, alone or with hydrochlorothiazide, versus nifedipine GITS in patients with essential hypertension. *Clin. Ther.* 18(3):411-28.

[11] Saito I, Fujikawa K, Saruta T. Cost-effectiveness analysis: controlled-release nifedipine and valsartan combination therapy in patients with essential hypertension: the adalat CR and valsartan cost-effectiveness combination (ADVANCE-Combi) study. *Hypertens. Res.* 2008;31(7): 1399-405.

[12] Study O. Efficacy and Tolerability of Long-Acting Nifedipine GITS / OROS Monotherapy or Combination Therapy in Hypertensive Patients. 2011:631-643.

[13] Pontremoli R, Leoncini G, Parodi A. Use of nifedipine in the treatment of hypertension. *Expert Rev. Cardiovasc. Ther.* 2005;3(1):43-50.

[14] Matsuoka H. [STONE study and INSIGHT study: efficacy of nifedipine in the prevention of cardiovascular disease in hypertensive patients]. *Drugs* 2006;66 Spec No(1):13-5.

[15] Mancia G, Brown M, Castaigne A, et al. Outcomes with nifedipine GITS or Co-amilozide in hypertensive diabetics and nondiabetics in Intervention as a Goal in Hypertension (INSIGHT). *Hypertension* 2003;41(3):431-6.

[16] Hall WD, Reed JW, Flack JM, et al. Comparison of the efficacy of dihydropyridine calcium channel blockers in African American patients with hypertension. ISHIB Investigators Group. International Society on Hypertension in Blacks. *Arch. Intern. Med.* 1998;158(18):2029-34.

[17] Weir MR, Sugimotto D, Gray J et al. Safety and efficacy of once daily captopril plus hydrochlorthiazide vs Nifedipine GITS in black patients with mild to moderate hypertension. *Am J Ther* 1996 : 3: 811-7.

[18] Derosa G, Cicero AFG, Bertone G, et al. Comparison of the effects of telmisartan and nifedipine gastrointestinal therapeutic system on blood pressure control, glucose metabolism, and the lipid profile in patients with type 2 diabetes mellitus and mild hypertension: a 12-month, randomized, doubl. *Clin. Ther.* 2004;26(8):1228-36.

[19] Crepaldi G, Carraro A, Brocco E, et al. Hypertension and non-insulin-dependent diabetes. A comparison between an angiotensin-converting

enzyme inhibitor and a calcium antagonist. *Acta Diabetol.* 1995;32(3):203-8.

[20] Savonitto S, Ardissino D, Egstrup K, et al. Combination therapy with metoprolol and nifedipine versus monotherapy in patients with stable angina pectoris results of the international multicenter angina exercise (IMAGE) study. *J. Am. Coll. Cardiol.* 1996;27(2):311-316.

[21] PRESERVE trial surprises with unexpected results on LV hypertrophy reduction with calcium channel blockers. *Cardiovasc. J. S. Afr.* 13(1):37-8.

[22] Schulte KL, Meyer-Sabellek W, Liederwald K, et al. Relation of regression of left ventricular hypertrophy to changes in ambulatory blood pressure after long-term therapy with perindopril versus nifedipine. *Am. J. Cardiol.* 1992;70(4):468-73.

[23] Shimokawa H. ACTION Study : Efficacy of Nifedipine in Preventing Cardiovascular Disease in. 2006;(1):10-12.

[24] Sierra C, Coca A. The ACTION study: nifedipine in patients with symptomatic stable angina and hypertension. *Expert Rev. Cardiovasc. Ther.* 2008;6(8):1055-62.

[25] Simon a, Gariépy J, Moyse D, et al. Differential effects of nifedipine and co-amilozide on the progression of early carotid wall changes. *Circulation* 2001;103(24):2949-54.

[26] Walker JM, Curry P V, Bailey AE, et al. A comparison of nifedipine once daily (Adalat LA), isosorbide mononitrate once daily, and isosorbide dinitrate twice daily in patients with chronic stable angina. *Int. J. Cardiol.* 1996;53(2):117-26.

[27] Yui Y. [JMIC-B study and its sub-analyses: effect of nifedipine in Japanese hypertensive patients with coronary artery disease]. *Drugs* 2006;66 Spec No(1):25-7.

[28] Thompson AE, Shea B, Welch V, et al. Calcium-channel blockers for Raynaud's phenomenon in systemic sclerosis. *Arthritis Rheum 2001;44:1841-7.*

[29] Hasebe N. [NICE-Combi study: effect of nifedipine in combination with an angiotensin II receptor blocker on BP control and renal protection]. *Drugs* 2006;66 Spec No(1):16-8.

[30] Yoshino G. [J-MIND study: effect of nifedipine on renal function in Japanese hypertensive patients with diabetes mellitus]. *Drugs* 2006;66 Spec No:22-24.

[31] ACOG practice bulletin no. 127: Management of preterm labor. *Obstet. Gynecol.* 2012;119(6):1308-17.

[32] Aguilar HN, Mitchell BF. Physiological pathways and molecular mechanisms regulating uterine contractility. *Hum. Reprod. Update* 16(6):725-44.

[33] Flenady V, Wojcieszek AM, Papatsonis DNM, et al. Calcium channel blockers for inhibiting preterm labour and birth. *Cochrane database Syst. Rev.* 2014;6:CD002255.

[34] Van Veen AJ, Pelinck MJ, van Pampus MG, et al. Severe hypotension and fetal death due to tocolysis with nifedipine. *BJOG* 2005;112(4): 509-10.

[35] Koontz SL, Friedman SA, Schwartz ML. Symptomatic hypocalcemia after tocolytic therapy with magnesium sulfate and nifedipine. *Am. J. Obstet. Gynecol.* 2004;190(6):1773-6.

[36] Cornette J, Duvekot J, Roos-Hesselink J, et al. Maternal and fetal haemodynamic effects of nifedipine in normotensive pregnant women. *BJOG* 2010.

[37] Beach MA, Mauro LS. Pharmacologic expulsive treatment of ureteral calculi. *Ann. Pharmacother.* 2006;40(7-8):1361-8.

[38] Deshwal R, Iqbal M, Basnet S. Nifedipine for the treatment of high altitude pulmonary edema. *Wilderness Environ. Med.* 2012;23(1):7-10.

In: Pulmonary Arterial Hypertension … ISBN: 978-1-63482-594-8
Editor: Victoria Estrada

Chapter IV

Nifedipine's Role in the Management of Pulmonary Hypertension

Raj Parikh, MD
Department of Internal Medicine,
Rush University Medical Center,
Chicago, IL, US

Abstract

Nifedipine has served as one of many advanced therapy options in the treatment of pulmonary hypertension. In comparison to other classes of agents, nifedipine has less adverse effects and can prove to be a preferred option when patients are requiring advanced therapy. In this chapter, the author summarizes the primary and advanced therapeutic options in the management of pulmonary hypertension. Then, the authors focuses on the role of nifedipine with highlights from research studies that have examined the benefits of nifedipine in varying classes of pulmonary hypertension. Lastly, the concept for future studies to examine nifedipine's role in comparison to other advanced therapy agents is introduced and the potential advantages are highlighted.

Introduction to Pulmonary Hypertension

Pulmonary hypertension (PH) is a disorder of the pulmonary arteries that is characterized by an elevated mean pulmonary arterial pressure (mPAP). It can be a progressive and debilitating disease, with 5-year survival rates often as low as 60% [1]. PH is sub-divided into specific categories based on its causes.. The World Health Organization (WHO) classification for PH consists of 5 groups [2]. Group 1 includes connective tissue diseases, idiopathic PH, and pulmonary arterial hypertension (PAH), group 2 includes PH secondary to left heart disease, group 3 consists of PH secondary to primary pulmonary disorders, group 4 includes PH secondary to chronic thromboembolic disease, and group 5 focuses on multifactorial mechanisms, such as sarcoidosis and myeloproliferative disorders.

Treatment of Pulmonary Hypertension

Since progressive disease may be refractory to therapy, early diagnosis and treatment of PH is highly recommended [3]. PH therapy is commonly referred to as primary and advanced. Primary therapy generally focuses on treating the underlying causes of PH while advanced therapy is directed towards reducing hypertension in the pulmonary vasculature. Common agents that comprise primary therapy for PH include diuretics, anticoagulants, digoxin, supplemental oxygen, and exercise through pulmonary rehabilitation. These above mechanisms have a role in treating PH regardless of the WHO classification.

The role of diuretics is to treat fluid retention and by doing so, diminish hepatic congestion and peripheral edema [4]. Moreover, PH patients are at increased risk for thromboembolic diseases because of limited pulmonary blood flow caused by increased afterload. Anticoagulants, such as warfarin, are commonly used in the therapy of PH, especially for WHO group 1 and 4 patients, and have also shown to have mortality benefits [5, 6]. Digoxin, meanwhile, has a role in improving right ventricular ejection fraction in patients with WHO group 2 and 3 [7]. Supplemental oxygen is indicated when patients with PH have documented hypoxemia [8]. Lastly, pulmonary rehabilitation has shown beneficial effects for PH patients as well [9, 10]. Among these benefits, improvements in functional exercise capacity and peak oxygen consumption have been seen.

Right heart catheterization (RHC) is the gold standard for diagnosis of PH [11]. Results from RHC will show an elevated mPAP, generally greater than 25 mmHg.

Advanced therapy for PH is only administered following completion of a diagnostic RHC. Advanced therapy includes the use of prostanoids, endothelin receptor antagonists (ERAs), phosphodiesterase 5 (PDE5) inhibitors, guanylate cyclase (GC) stimulants, and calcium channel blockers (CCBs).

Vasoreactivity Testing

Specific to WHO group 1 PH patients, the RHC is accompanied by vasoreactivity testing. This involves evaluating patients and determining whether their degree of PH would be responsive to CCBs, which are less toxic than other agents used for advanced therapy [12]. During vasoreactivity testing, a short-acting vasodilator, such as inhaled nitric oxide, adenosine, or prostacyclins, is administered and its effects on hemodynamics is then measured [13]. A positive test is denoted by a decrease in mPAP by at least 10 mmHg without significant changes seen in systemic blood pressure and an increase or unchanged cardiac output. If the vasoreactivity tests fail to show a decrease in mPAP, then advanced therapy agents, not including CCBs, are often the next step in therapy.

Prostanoids

Prostanoids include epoprostenol, which has been shown to improve survival in WHO group 1 patients [14]. Additionally, epoprostenol has improved hemodynamic parameters and functional capacity in all WHO groups [15]. Another prostanoid, treprostinil, has also shown improvements in hemodynamics, exercise capacity, and overall symptoms in WHO group 1 patients [16-18].

Endothelin Receptor Antagonists

Endothelin-1 is a vasoconstrictor agent that exists in high concentrations in PH patients while playing a primary role in inducing increased afterload in the pulmonary vasculature [19]. ERAs, including both non-selective and selective agents, serve to decrease endothelin-1 concentrations. Non-selective agents include bosentan and macitentan while selective agents include ambrisentan and sitaxsentant. Bosentan has been shown to delay clinical worsening and improve exercise tolerance and hemodynamics in patients with idiopathic PH. Futhermore, the BREATHE-1 trial depicted the role of Bosentan in improving symptoms and six-minute walk distance in patients with severe WHO group 1 PH. A meta-analysis consisting of 1471 patients delineated the beneficial effects of other ERAs in patients with PAH, which included improved exercise capacity, decreased dyspnea, and improved hemodynamic parameters as noted by RHC [20]. Other trials looking at the use of selective ERAs in patients with WHO groups 2, 3, and 4 were also able to show improved exercise tolerance, quality of life, and hemodynamics [21-22].

Phosphodiesterase 5 Inhibitors

PDE5 inhibitors include sildenafil, tadalafil, and vardenafil. The SUPER-1 trial examined the effects of sildenafil on patients with WHO group 1 PH and an improvement in hemodynamics and six-minute walk distances was seen [23]. The PHIRST trial showed similar effects with tadalafil [24].

Guanylate Cyclase Stimulants

GC stimulants work directly to stimulate nitric oxide receptors as well as increase the sensitivity of the receptors to nitric oxide. This dual effect was witnessed in the CHEST-1 trial, which examined the role of an oral GC stimulant, in WHO group 4 patients [25]. Another trial, PATENT-1, looked at WHO group 2 and 3 patients and results were significant for an improvement in exercise capacity, as was measured by the six-minute walk test [26].

Nifedipine Therapy for Pulmonary Hypertension

PH patients who undergo RHC and pass vasoreactivity testing are candidates to be treated with CCBs. CCBs, such as diltiazem and nifedipine, have proven to be effective therapeutic options for PH because of multiple mechanisms. CCBs show an ability to inhibit hypoxic vasoconstriction in animal models [27].

Moreover, in cases of idiopathic PH, voltage-gated potassium channels are often down regulated [28]. This down regulation results in membrane depolarization and the subsequent release of intracellular calcium, which then directly plays a role in increased contraction and proliferation of pulmonary artery smooth muscle cells [29-30]. Therefore, CCBs help decrease this high concentration of calcium and essentially, prevent pulmonary artery vasoconstriction.

The first case report of nifedipine being used to treat PH was described in 1980, where an improvement in exercise capacity and symptoms was seen in a patient after 3 months of treatment [31].

Another study showed that nifedipine was able to increase CO and therefore, reduce pulmonary vascular resistance [32]. Furthermore, research indicated that high-dose nifedipine also directly effected pulmonary hemodynamics, including decreasing mPAP [33].

The largest prospective study examining the effects of nifedipine on idiopathic PH consisted of 71 patients with results significant for decreased mPAP and improved survival in the experimental arm of the investigation [34]. Outside of idiopathic PH, patients with PH secondary to connective tissue diseases have also shown to have improvements in hemodynamic parameters, including decreases in mPAP, with administration of nifedipine [35].

Conclusion

There are several therapeutic options for advanced therapy in PH patients. However, pending vasoreactivity testing results during RHC, CCBs prove to be the least toxic of these advanced therapy agents. Prostanoids, ERAs, PDE5 inhibitors, and GC stimulants all come with their share of adverse side effects. On the other hand, CCBs such as nifedipine do not have a history of producing severe adverse effects in patients with PH or in patients requiring the use of CCBs for other causes.

Thus, it is not surprising that CCBs have a long history of beneficial use in treating PH. However, comparison of different CCBs in treating PH has yet to be studied. Furthermore, examining the use of nifedipine in comparison to other advanced therapy options in PH patients has not been accomplished either. While CCBs such as nifedipine have been thoroughly researched, the absence of such comparison studies limits the evidence to prove nifedipine's worth in PH therapy.

Future research should focus on comparing advanced therapy options in PH patients as well as analyzing adverse effects of CCBs versus the other classes.

References

[1] McLaughlin, V., Presberg, K., et al. (Apr. 22, 2006). Prognosis of pulmonary arterial hypertension. *Chest,* 126: 78-92.

[2] Simonneau G., Robbins I., Beghetti M., et al. Updated clinical classification of pulmonary hypertension. *J. Am. Coll. Cardiol.,* 2009; 54:S43-S54.

[3] Galiè N., Rubin Lj., Hoeper M., et al. Treatment of patients with mildly symptomatic pulmonary arterial hypertension with bosentan (EARLY study): a double-blind, randomised controlled trial. *Lancet,* 2008; 371: 2093.

[4] Galiè N., Hoeper M. M., Humbert M., et al. Guidelines for the diagnosis and treatment of pulmonary hypertension: the Task Force for the Diagnosis and Treatment of Pulmonary Hypertension of the European Society of Cardiology (ESC) and the European Respiratory Society (ERS), endorsed by the International Society of Heart and Lung Transplantation (ISHLT). *Eur. Heart J.,* 2009; 30:2493.

[5] Olsson K. M., Delcroix M., Ghofrani H. A., et al. Anticoagulation and survival in pulmonary arterial hypertension: results from the Comparative, Prospective Registry of Newly Initiated Therapies for Pulmonary Hypertension (COMPERA). *Circulation,* 2014; 129:57.

[6] Johnson S. R., Mehta S., Granton J. T. Anticoagulation in pulmonary arterial hypertension: a qualitative systematic review. *Eur. Respir. J.,* 2006; 28:999.

[7] Mathur P. N., Powles P., Pugsley S. O., et al. Effect of digoxin on right ventricular function in severe chronic airflow obstruction. A controlled clinical trial. *Ann. Intern. Med.,* 1981; 95:283.

[8] McLaughlin V. V., Archer S. L., Badesch D. B., et al. ACCF/AHA 2009 expert consensus document on pulmonary hypertension: a report of the

American College of Cardiology Foundation Task Force on Expert Consensus Documents and the American Heart Association: developed in collaboration with the American College of Chest Physicians, American Thoracic Society, Inc., and the Pulmonary Hypertension Association. *Circulation*, 2009; 119:2250.

[9] Mereles D., Ehlken N., Kreuscher S., et al. Exercise and respiratory training improve exercise capacity and quality of life in patients with severe chronic pulmonary hypertension. *Circulation,* 2006; 114:1482.

[10] Weinstein A. A., Chin L. M., Keyser R. E., et al. Effect of aerobic exercise training on fatigue and physical activity in patients with pulmonary arterial hypertension. *Respir. Med.,* 2013; 107:778.

[11] Simonneau G., Gatzoulis M. A., Adatia I., et al. Updated clinical classification of pulmonary hypertension. *J. Am. Coll. Cardiol.*, 2013; 62:D34.

[12] Taichman D. B., Ornelas J., Chung L., et al. Pharmacologic therapy for pulmonary arterial hypertension in adults: CHEST guideline and expert panel report. *Chest,* 2014; 146:449.

[13] Galiè N., Corris P. A., Frost A., et al. Updated treatment algorithm of pulmonary arterial hypertension. *J. Am. Coll. Cardiol.*, 2013; 62:D60.

[14] Barst R. J., Rubin L. J., Long W. A., et al. A comparison of continuous intravenous epoprostenol (prostacyclin) with conventional therapy for primary pulmonary hypertension. *N. Engl. J. Med.,* 1996; 334:296.

[15] McLaughlin V. V., Genthner D. E., Panella M. M., et al. Compassionate use of continuous prostacyclin in the management of secondary pulmonary hypertension: a case series. *Ann. Intern. Med.*, 1999; 130: 740.

[16] Tapson V. F., Gomberg-Maitland M., McLaughlin V. V., et al. Safety and efficacy of IV treprostinil for pulmonary arterial hypertension: a prospective, multicenter, open-label, 12-week trial. *Chest,* 2006; 129: 683.

[17] Simonneau G., Barst R. J., Galie N., et al. Continuous subcutaneous infusion of treprostinil, a prostacyclin analogue, in patients with pulmonary arterial hypertension: a double-blind, randomized, placebo-controlled trial. *Am. J. Respir. Crit. Care Med.,* 2002; 165:800.

[18] Benza R. L., Tapson V. F., Gomberg-Maitland M., et al. One-year experience with intravenous treprostinil for pulmonary arterial hypertension. *J. Heart Lung Transplant.*, 2013; 32:889.

[19] Channick R. N., Sitbon O., Barst R. J., et al. Endothelin receptor antagonists in pulmonary arterial hypertension. *J. Am. Coll. Cardiol.,* 2004; 43:62S.

[20] Liu C., Chen J., Gao Y., et al. Endothelin receptor antagonists for pulmonary arterial hypertension. *Cochrane Database Syst. Rev.*, 2013; 2:CD004434.

[21] Galié N., Badesch D., Oudiz R., et al. Ambrisentan therapy for pulmonary arterial hypertension. *J. Am. Coll. Cardiol.*, 2005; 46:529.

[22] Oudiz R. J., Galiè N., Olschewski H., et al. Long-term ambrisentan therapy for the treatment of pulmonary arterial hypertension. *J. Am. Coll. Cardiol.*, 2009; 54:1971.

[23] Galiè N., Ghofrani H. A., Torbicki A., et al. Sildenafil citrate therapy for pulmonary arterial hypertension. N. Engl. J. Med., 2005; 353:2148.

[24] Galiè N., Brundage B. H., Ghofrani H. A., et al. Tadalafil therapy for pulmonary arterial hypertension. *Circulation,* 2009; 119:2894.

[25] Ghofrani H. A., D'Armini A. M., Grimminger F., et al. Riociguat for the treatment of chronic thromboembolic pulmonary hypertension. *N. Engl. J. Med.,* 2013; 369:319.

[26] Ghofrani H. A., Galiè N., Grimminger F., et al. Riociguat for the treatment of pulmonary arterial hypertension. *N. Engl. J. Med.,* 2013; 369:330.

[27] Palevsky H. I., Schloo B. L., Pietra G. G., et al. Primary pulmonary hypertension. Vascular structure, morphometry, and responsiveness to vasodilator agents. *Circulation,* 1989; 80:1207-1221.

[28] Yuan J. X., Aldinger A. M., Juhaszova M., et al. Dysfunctional voltage-gated K+ channels in pulmonary artery smooth muscle cells of patients with primary pulmonary hypertension. *Circulation*, 1998; 98: 1400-1406.

[29] Pollock D. M., Keith T. L., Highsmith R. F. Endothelin receptors and calcium signaling. *FASEB J.,* 1995;9:1196-1204.

[30] Corbin J. D. Mechanisms of action of PDE5 inhibition in erectile dysfunction. *Int. J. Impot. Res.,* 2004;16(Suppl. 1):S4-7.

[31] Camerini F., Alberti E., Klugmann S., et al. Primary pulmonary hypertension: effects of nifedipine. *Br. Heart J.,* 1980; 44:352-356.

[32] Rubin L. J., Nicod P., Hillis L. D., et al. Treatment of primary pulmonary hypertension with nifedipine. A hemodynamic and scintigraphic evaluation. *Ann. Intern. Med.,* 1983;99:433-438.

[33] Rich S., Brundage B. H. High-dose calcium channel-blocking therapy for primary pulmonary hypertension: evidence for long-term reduction

in pulmonary arterial pressure and regression of right ventricular hypertrophy. *Circulation,* 1987; 76:135-141.

[34] Rich S., Kaufmann E., Levy P. S. The effect of high doses of calcium-channel blockers on survival in primary hypertension. *N. Engl. J. Med.,* 1992; 327:76-81. Nootens M., Kaufmann E., Rich S. Short-term effectiveness of nifedipine in secondary pulmonary hypertension. *Am. J. Cardiol.,* 1993; 71:1475-1476.

[35] Alpert M. A., Pressly T. A., Mukerji V., et al. Acute and long-term effects of nifedipine on pulmonary and systemic hemodynamics in patients with pulmonary hypertension associated with diffuse systemic sclerosis, the CREST syndrome and mixed connective tissue disease. *Am. J. Cardiol.,* 1991; 68:1687-1691.

In: Pulmonary Arterial Hypertension … ISBN: 978-1-63482-594-8
Editor: Victoria Estrada

Chapter V

Nifedipine Controlled Release Systems Based on Inorganic Materials: A Review from the Start of the New Millenium to Present Date

Inês J. Marques [1]***, Pedro D. Vaz*** [2] ***and Carla D. Nunes*** [1]
[1]CQB, Departamento de Química e Bioquímica, Faculdade de Ciências da Universidade de Lisboa, Portugal
[2]ISIS Facility, Rutherford Appleton Laboratory, Chilton, Didcot, Oxfordshire OX11 0QX, United Kingdom

Abstract

Calcium channel blockers (CCBs) are widely used for the management of hypertension and angina. Prescription drug sales of CCBs in the United States accounted for US$11.6 billion in 2004, ranking them as the eighth largest drug class in prescription sales. Within this class, Nifedipine, a potent dihydropyridine agent, is widely prescribed accounting for a large share of the annual sales volume.

Despite all benefits and versatility presented by such drug (among other counterparts) there are a few drawbacks concerning its use. The main problem with such drug is its low solubility which limits its bioavailability, making it perform less efficiently towards therapeutic use than it can. To circumvent this many research is dedicated to this issue in order to find new polymorphic forms of the drug leading to higher solubility and ultimately to higher bioavailability. On the other hand research is also conducted to develop controlled drug delivery systems bearing in mind that these can lead to better release kinetics, to better patient wellbeing and to better drug resistance and stability to aggressive environmental body conditions (gastric fluids, etc…). Due to confinement effects, such drug delivery systems can also lead to different crystallization forms of the immobilized drug which can lead to better solubility and bioavailability.

Recent years have experienced the development of new approaches to prepare such drug delivery systems based on inorganic matrix materials. Taking advantage of the porosity presented by such systems, drugs can be encapsulated becoming then protected and being ready for release.

This chapter lights up some recent advances on this niche research topic covering the most relevant advances in the timeframe between 2000 and the present date.

Introduction

Nifedipine (*Nif*), Figure 1, a potent dihydropyridine calcium-channel blocking (CCB) agent, is widely used for the treatment of hypertension and as antianginal agent (especially in Prinzmetal's angina) [1,2].

However, the bioavailability of *Nif* is relatively low after oral administration of crystalline form due to its limited solubility in water (ca. 20 μg mL^{-1}) [3–5]. Various oral formulations of *Nif* such as solid dispersions [6–9], inclusion complex [10], nanocrystal [11] and micronization of drug [12] were developed to improve the solubility and bioavailability of *Nif*. Furthermore, a prolonged action of *Nif* is another prime consideration for the effective treatment of hypertension, since *Nif* is rapidly eliminated from the plasma compartment and its antihypertensive action lasts only for a few hours [3–5].

Oral drug delivery systems have been widely accepted due to ease of administration, avoiding a chance of pain or infection possibly involved with needle-based injection [13,14]. Among diverse types of commercialized drug delivery products, more than half of them are designed for an oral administration route [15]. Most oral drug delivery systems were developed to sustain or delay drug release over time, hence leading to enhanced drug bioavailability as well as reduced side effects.

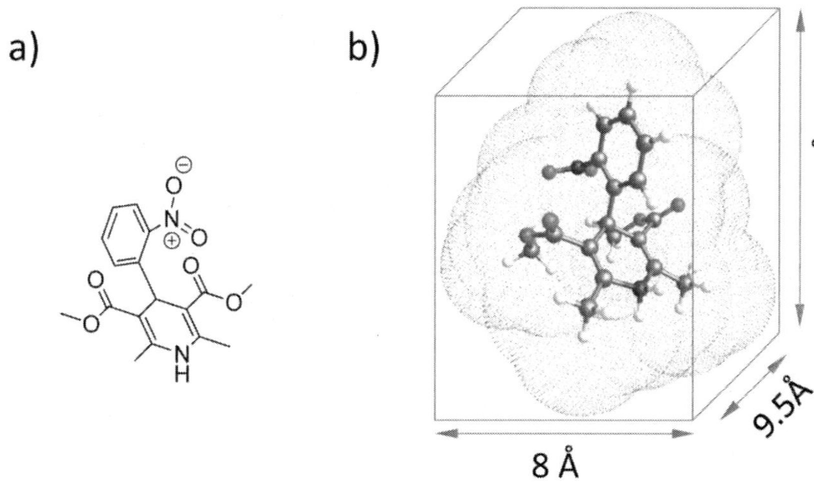

Figure 1. Schematic representation of a) nifedipine and b) 3D representation including the van der Waals radius fitted by a box showing its approximate dimensions.

In this context, inorganic materials serve this purpose quite well due to a good level of biocompatibility. Although their application to Nifedipine is limited, this chapter will give an updated view of the present state of the art. The following sections will devote to describe three major families of inorganic materials which were tested as delivery systems for *Nif.*

Calcium Phosphate Cement (CPC)

Calcium phosphate biomaterials can virtually all be classified as polycrystalline ceramics. These materials are formed by a process called sintering in which high temperatures (1100 – 1300 °C), pressures, and different apatites are used to yield the final product, calcium phosphates. Combining a given temperature, pressure, and different apatite sources has a detrimental effect on several properties of the final product. For example, pure hydroxyapatite (HA) is formed by using apatite with a Ca/P ratio of 1.7, whereas tricalciumphosphate (TCP) is formed by using apatite with a Ca/P ratio of 1.5.

When apatites with varying Ca/P ratios are sintered, different amounts of HA and TCP are formed in the final ceramic, yielding biphasic calcium phosphates (BCPs).

Sinteting parameters and techniques also determine the final residual microporosity [16]. The microporosity of the ceramics is due to cavities left between the sintered particles, being mostly biased by the crystallization of the apatite(s) used. Dense and porous ceramics are produced by different sintering techniques.

Calcium phosphate ceramics can dissolve across a full range of pH solutions, depending on their chemical composition. Especially in acidic environments calcium phosphate ceramics dissolve rapidly. The Ca/P ratio of the ceramic used is mostly important to this process. TCP (Ca/P < 1.67) dissolves 12.3 times faster than HA (Ca/P = 1.7) in acidic medium and 22.3 times faster than HA in basic medium [17]. Other properties of the biomaterial, i.e., porosity, crystallinity, and impurities of the biomaterial can influence this process.

The dissolution process results in an increase of the extra-cellular concentrations of calcium ($[Ca^{2+}]_{ec}$) and phosphorous ($[PO_4^{3-}]_{ec}$). The high $[Ca^{2+}]_{ec}$ and $[PO_4^{3-}]_{ec}$ leads to the precipitation of apatites on a ceramic substrate, forming a carbonate-apatite-crystal layer. The very strong interface between the material and bone is believed to be influenced by this crystal layer [16].

In addition, formation of apatite crystals at the surface of a ceramic stimulates the process of epitaxial crystal growth. HA, as stated before, has a low dissolution rate which results in almost direct bonding with bone and tissue components.

Self-setting type of calcium phosphate cement (CPC) was developed by Brown and Chow in 1986 on the basis of the solubility phase chart of calcium phosphate.

Nifedipine-containing calcium phosphate cement (CPC) was prepared by Suzuki *et al.* who studied drug release from CPC preparations using nifedipine (Nif) by three dissolution test methods, *i.e.* the shaking method (SK), Japanese Pharmacopoeia XIV (JPXIV) paddle method (PD), and JPXIV flow-through cell method (FT) [18].

The drug release from the planar surface of the homogeneous drug-loaded matrix system followed the Higuchi equation:

$$M(t) = \sqrt{\frac{D_i \varepsilon (2C_d - \varepsilon C_s) C_s t}{\tau}}$$

where $M(t)$ is the cumulative amount of drug released (until time t), D_i is the diffusion coefficient of the drug in the matrix, ε is the porosity of the matrix, C_d is the total concentration of the drug in the matrix, C_s is the solubility of the drug in the matrix and τ is the tortuosity of the capillary system.

Data show that excelent slow-release preparations of *Nif* are considered to be obtained by processing it as CPC. The Higuchi constant differed according to the *Nif* concentration in the matrix on the same test, the values of the parameters involved in dissolution (τ, ε, D_i, C_s) were constant under the conditions of Suzuki's *et al.* study. FT showed the most rapid dissolution and is considered to be advantageous for rapid evaluation of dissolution characteristics of the active drug from slowly dissolving slow-release preparations.

Porous Silicates

Porous inorganic solids, such as aero- and xerogels and zeolites, have found great utility due to their large internal surface area, arising from the presence of voids of controllable dimensions at the atomic, molecular, and nanometer scales. With increasing environmental concerns worldwide, nanoporous materials have become more and more important and useful for the separation of polluting species and the recovery of useful ones. This works for small molecules (having kinetic diameter below 1 nm), but in a reaction reactants many times have dimensions above those making impossible to access the pores.

In the early 1990's new families of mesoporous materials (with pore diameters ranging between 2 and 50 nm) known as KSW-1 [19], FSM-16 [20], and M41S [21], were discovered, opening new possibilities to new applications involving large molecules. The silicate wall of the pores is amorphous. Mesoporous silicates, such as MCM-41 and SBA-15 (the most common mesoporous silicates), are porous silicates with huge surface areas (normally $\geq$1000 m^2/g), large pore sizes (2 nm $\leq$ size $\leq$ 20 nm) and ordered arrays of cylindrical mesopores with very regular pore morphology, as evidenced in Figure 2.

The most popular family of mesoporous materials, and the main contributor to the development of the chemistry of mesoporous materials, was discovered by researchers of the Mobil Oil Corporation in 1992 [19,20]. This family of materials is known as M41S and is composed by three materials, MCM-41, MCM-48 and MCM-50, having structures with hexagonal, cubic and lamellar arrays of the pores, respectively. Among them, MCM-41 is, by far, the most used and studied. Since then many other materials have been developed with similar engineered properties, such as SBA-15 and HMS among others.

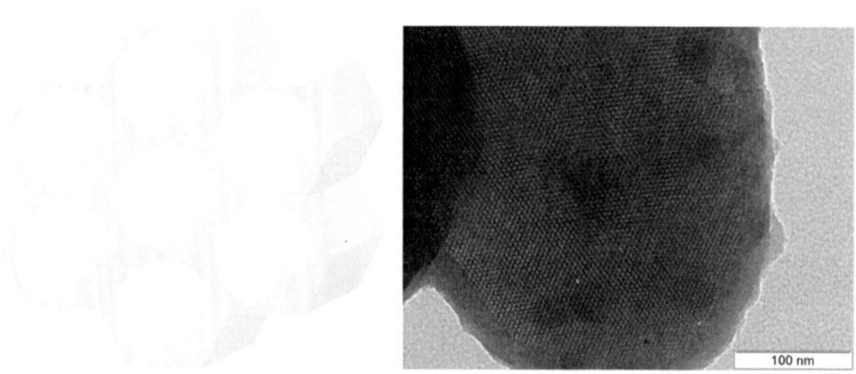

Figure 2. Schematic representation of the hexagonal array of pores in MCM-41 (left) and TEM micrograph of a MCM-41 sample (right).

Compared to previous systems prior to the discovery of the M41s family, the few known mesoporous materials were characterized by irregular size distribution and spacing of the pores. In contrast, the M41s materials presented a narrow pore size distribution and a hexagonal array of the pores. These materials have important properties, such as a high surface area and a high density of silanol groups (Si-OH) at its surface which make these materials suitable to promote the immobilization of large molecules inside their pores. These properties help to promote the immobilization of relatively large molecules inside their pores, though care must be taken to prevent pore blocking. MCM-41 also proved to be very good for hosting molecules of several sizes, shapes and functionalities [22,23]. This silicate-based material has been the aim of many biological studies concerning its use as drug delivery systems [24,25]. However recent studies have shown that MCM-41 lead to marginal toxic phenotypes in some cells which can be classified as early response of cells towards an environmental stressor [26].

During the last few years, porous materials have met important breakthrough by experiencing new applications especially in drug delivery systems. As part of this strategy, encapsulating poorly soluble drugs in mesoporous silicates is an emerging strategy to improve drug dissolution.

A promising technique for preparation of controlled delivery systems is the sol–gel procedure [27,28], which involves the manufacture of an inorganic matrix through the gelation of a colloidal suspension (sol) at low temperature and in mild conditions. This technique also allows incorporation of highly sensitive molecules, like proteins and peptides into the gel [29,30]. This technique offers new possibilities for embedding organic compounds within silica and other modified inorganic oxides (Sol-gel carriers). The technology is simple and versatile, with the oxide matrix being cheap, inert and stable to light and heat without being hazardous to humans or the environment [31]. Silica-based materials produced using the sol–gel technique has been shown to be biocompatible *in vivo* because these materials are readily degradable inside the body. Such systems cause no adverse tissue reactions because they degrade into $Si(OH)_4$, which is easily eliminated from the body through the kidneys [32].

Nifedipine (*Nif*), a CCB agent, has a poor aqueous solubility, resulting in low and often irregular bioavailability. However, if one attains a sustained release of *Nif*, for example, by incorporating it into a porous insoluble matrix, one could achieve an increased effectiveness with fewer side effects, as shown in the case of intravenous infusion. Uroŝ Maver *et al.* studied the correlations between the morphological features and release properties of *Nif* incorporated into porous silica. These correlations should give a solid background for designing specific systems for intravenous infusion of *Nif* [33]. They achieved a predetermined plasma concentration that can be maintained via the subsequent diffusion of the incorporated drug out of the insoluble matrix. Alternatively, one could use such composites to suppress the dissolution and absorption rate in cases where too high rates could lead to toxic side effects.

Nifedipine immobilized into a modified silica matrix by the sol-gel technique allows its releasing behavior to be controlled to a high degree. The release rate is proportional to temperature and is increased by the addition of penetration agents such as sorbitol, but is inversely proportional to particle size and is decreased by modification of the silica matrix with methyltriethoxysilane or polyethyleneglycol. It is presumed that the drug is dispersed in the gel matrix and that diffusion occurs through solvent-filled capillary channels [34].

H.Böttcher *et al.* showed that the releasing behavior of *Nif* from the silica matrix can be controlled to a high degree by the sol-gel technique. The rate of liberation of nifedipine from the composite is inversely proportional to the mean grain size, *d* [31]. The smaller the grain size, the greater the release rate, as driven by the surface-to-bulk ratio. Before release of the drug can occur, it must diffuse from within the increasingly large grain volume to the composite surface.

The releasing rate of nifedipine is also influenced by chemical or physical changes to the silica matrix. One possible chemical change is the modification by organofunctional metal alkoxides or trialkoxysilanes during the sol preparation, such as co-hydrolysis of $Si(OEt)_4$ with $MeSi(OEt)_3$. Addition of other low or high molecular weight sol-soluble additives (sorbitol, polyethylene-glycol) also influence that property. In this way it is possible to produce composites with uniform drug release profiles over a long period of time and able to tune the releasing behavior to the pharmacokinetic demands [33].

Finding thermodynamic criteria that must be satisfied in order to prevent formation of crystalline state of drugs within a confined space is another important thing to pay attention. Some studies state that there exists a critical pore radius of a host below which the entrapped substance will solidify in an amorphous form. There also exists a critical pore radius below which the entrapped amorphous solid will not be able to crystallize. Specifically, incorporation of *Nif* into a silica xerogel with an average pore diameter of about 2.5 nm produces and stabilizes its amorphous form. The confined amorphous *Nif* is effectively protected against crystallization within the temperature range in which *Nif* itself is stable. Entrapment of drugs into solid nanoporous carriers could be regarded as a potentially useful and simple method for production and/or stabilization of non-crystalline forms of a wide range of drugs [35].

A study by Van Speybroeck *et al.* evaluated the applicability of the ordered mesoporous silicate SBA-15 as an excipient to enhance dissolution, for a test series of 10 poorly soluble compounds with a high degree of physicochemical diversity [36]. All SBA-15 formulations tested exhibited an enhanced dissolution as compared to their corresponding crystalline materials, and the high pharmaceutical performance of all formulations was retained during the 6 months storage period. The results of their study suggest that encapsulation in SBA-15 can be applied as a dissolution-enhancing formulation approach for a very wide variety of poorly soluble drugs.

It has been reported that physically mixing hydrophobic drugs with mesoporous silicates can already induce a high degree of interaction. Nifedipine has also been reported to benefit from adsorption onto high surface area silica-based carriers [37].

In that work *Nif* was released to 80% of drug loading within the first 5 min of the experiment. This rapid release arises from the fast dissolution of the confined material, followed by a quick diffusion into the bulk medium. Drug release was not slower for the larger molecules of the test series, indicating that the pore diameter of SBA-15 is sufficiently wide as to allow for a relatively unhindered diffusion of all test compounds.

Encapsulation in SBA-15confirmed that can be applied as a dissolution-enhancing formulation approach for a very wide variety of poorly soluble drugs. This shows great promise for the future, as every dissolution-enhancing formulation approach used nowadays is known to depend on the active compound's physicochemical profile.

It is clear that encapsulation in SBA-15 constitutes a potentially great expansion of the formulation scientist's toolbox to overcome dissolution-limited bioavailability.

Clays

Clays can be described as two-dimensional materials, since they are formed by layers of double hydroxides, and allow the intercalation of other species between them [38].

The importance of these materials is based on their ability to retain chemical species with electrical charges compatible to those of the layers. This can expand or contract the dimension along the basal axis (normally perpendicular to the layers), while the general structure is maintained (also called topotactic reaction). Layered lattices for intercalation reactions are described as two-dimensional (2D) because they are formed by layered units (layers), stacked along the basal direction. The bonds in the layers are covalent and the stacking is held by weak interactions such as van der Waals forces for neutral layers, and electrostatic forces for charged ones [39-41]. Nanocomposite materials reinforced with layered fillers in polymers are termed one-dimensional because only one dimension of the layer is in the nanometric range [42]. Many studies have been carried out on the subgroup of the anion-exchanging layered materials, especially on layered double hydroxides, focusing on their physicochemical properties, surface modification reactions and applications [43-48].

Cationic clays comprise, among others, smectites (which belong to the group of layered aluminosilicates, including two-dimensional phyllosilicates) such as montmorillonite (MMT), hectorite [49,50], and mica-type layered silicates. These materials find wide practical application, primarily by their well-pronounced intercalation properties. Clays are phyllosilicates or layered silicates with a layer lattice structure in which two-dimensional oxoanions are separated by layers of hydrated cations. The oxygen atoms define upper and lower sheets enclosing tetrahedral sites and a central sheet having the brucite or gibbsite structure enclosing octahedral sites. Smectites have two tetrahedral sheets (T) around the central octahedral sheet (O) in each layer, hence the name 2:1 phyllosilicate, Figure 3.

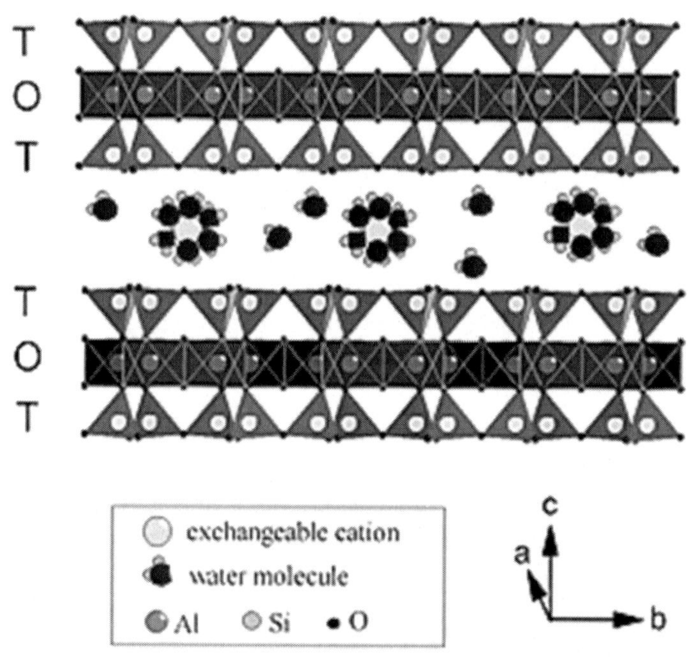

Figure 3. Layered 2:1 tetrahedral-octahedral-tetrahedral (TOT) structure of a smectite clay.

These layers have charge excess resulting from isomorphous substitutions (e.g Si^{4+} by Al^{3+} at tetrahedral sites or Al^{3+} by Mg^{2+} at octahedral sites). As such, these negatively charged layers are balanced by exchangeable hydrated interlayer cations such as Na^{+}, K^{+} or Ca^{2+}. The charge excess and its origin (octahedral versus tetrahedral) results in different physical and chemical properties, *e. g.*, thermal stability and swelling behavior. There are two ways by which the neutral layers of these minerals can be rendered negatively charged to obtain cationic clays:

1) By partial isomorphous substitution of Si^{IV} ions by M^{III} ions – usually Al – in the tetrahedral layers to give a layer composition of $[Mg_6(Si_{8-x}M^{III}_x)O_{20}(OH)_4]^{x-}$ or $[Al_4(Si_{8-x}M^{III}_x)O_{20}(OH)_4]^{x-}$.
2) By partial isomorphous substitution of Mg^{II} ions by M^I ions (in the case of talc) or Al^{III} ions by M^{II} ions (in the case of pyrophyllite) in the octahedral layers to give a layer composition of $[(Mg_{6-x}M^I_x)Si_8O_{20}(OH)_4]^{x-}$ or $[(Al_{4-x}M^{II}_x)Si_8O_{20}(OH)_4]^{x-}$.

Layer charges related to tetrahedral substitutions lead to a localized charge distribution, while layer charges related to octahedral substitutions are more distributed over the complete oxygen framework [51]. For instance in talc, the central plane of octahedral sites is occupied completely by Mg^{2+} ions, and in pyrophyllite, two-thirds of the octahedral sites are occupied by Al^{3+} ions.

In all these cases, the negative charge is compensated by the inclusion of positive ions in the interlayer region, which determines the classification as cationic clays. Intercalated cations are often hydrated leading to swelling of the material. The cationic clays exhibit wide compositional flexibility with x values ranging from 0.4 to 2.0. When x is in the $0.4 < x < 1.2$ range, the intercalated cations are exchangeable. However, when the extent of substitution is high $x = 2$ it leads to micas which do not exhibit cation exchange [52].

For instance montmorillonite-K10 is a bio inert clay mineral with fine grain and large interlayer- planar spacing in the 001 plane with a superior capability to intercalate large molecules into this space [53]. The interlayer-spacing depends much on conditions, becoming more open in basic medium, especially at pH values above 11 [54]. Although montmorillonite is an aluminosilicate, there is evidence that it is nearly non-toxic to living organisms [55] and the European Food & Safety Agency (EFSA) has recently approved its use as a food additive [56].

Clay characterization is a very important area relying on the use of spectroscopic techniques traditionally linked to solid-state and materials chemistry, such as solid-state NMR, vibrational (FTIR and Raman) and electronic (UV-Vis) spectroscopy, electron microscopy (SEM and TEM) among others [57-59].

The case study of clay nanotubes for encapsulation and sustained release of drugs by Veerabadran *et al.* used 50-nm diameter halloysite clay nanotubules with 15 nm lumen for loading poorly soluble drugs and sustaining their release. Loading was optimized by varying pH and alcohol/water ratio in the solvent with a maximum drug loading of 12% v/v [60].

Biocompatibility of halloysite nanotubules makes this method a prospective drug delivery system.

Halloysite ($Al_2Si_2O_5(OH)_4{\cdot}2H_2O$) is a two-layered aluminosilicate which has a predominantly hollow tubular structure in the submicron range and is chemically similar to kaolin. Our interest in this chapter is to focus on the entrapment, storage, and subsequent release of Nifedipine (anti-anginal). To increase loading of this poor soluble drugs, they loaded it in water–alcohol mixtures (0, 10, and 50% ethanol). Halloysite is biocompatible, but its biodegradability is unclear; therefore, its usage in medicine for sustained drug release is feasible for dermatological and dental applications.

Nif release was found to be 25 times longer from the tubules than from the crystals and an initial burst within 10 min followed by a 6–10 hour release period could be observed [60].

In the next section the use of some of the above mentioned materials as matrices for *Nif* and the associated drug delivery performance will be discussed.

Comparing Virtues & Limitations of Different Matrices

Although immobilization of *Nif* (and other drugs) has been accomplished in many different materials as matrix, performance comparison is not straightforward and is lacking as well. Therefore a case study comparing different matrices for controlled release of *Nif* showing virtues and limitations of both the matrices will be presented.

The chosen materials to be used as matrices were montmorrilonite K10 clay (hereafter denoted as *K10*) and the mesoporous silicate MCM-41 (hereafter denoted as *MCM*).

Nifedipine (*Nif*) is isolated as 3,5-dimethyl 2,6-dimethyl-4-(2-nitrophenyl)-1,4-dihydropyridine-3,5-dicarboxylate in its hydrochloride form (see the structure in Figure 1). As a result it holds a positive charge which renders it the possibility of undergoing ion exchange in order to be immobilized inside the interlayer spacing of cationic clays, such as *K10*. In the case of *MCM*, it holds channels with silanol (Si–OH) groups at the surface, which are adequate to interact with functional groups of guest molecules and therefore being able to host *Nif* guest molecules inside its pores.

Characterization of the Materials

Nifedipine (*Nif*) was incorporated in montmorillonite (*K10*) and in MCM-41 (*MCM*), by mixing in dichloromethane a given amount of the matrix material (either K10 or MCM) with *Nif*, affording two composite materials designated as *K10nif* and *MCMnif*. From elemental analysis the *Nif* loading was found to reach 0.04 mol% and 0.07 mol % for *K10nif* and *MCMnif* respectively. This means that *K10nif* and *MCMnif* are formulated, respectively, as 138 mg_{Nif}/g_{K10} and 242 mg_{Nif}/g_{MCM}. The described drug loading process for the two materials was found to be reproducible by ±5%.

Characterization of the resulting drug loaded materials was accomplished by means of adequate spectroscopic techniques traditionally linked to solid-state and materials chemistry: vibrational (FTIR) and electronic (UV-Vis) spectroscopy, electron microscopy (SEM and TEM) and powder XRD.

The FTIR spectra of the composite materials (*K10nif* and *MCMnif*) as well as the vibrational spectrum of *Nif* are collected in Figure 4.

The spectra of both *K10nif* and *MCMnif* composite materials are dominated by modes from the matrix materials. For instance, $\nu_{O\text{–}H}$ modes present broad and intense bands assigned to hydrogen bonded hydroxyl groups, whereas bands in this region are indicative of free OH groups of the host matrices. Broad and very intense features corresponding to $\nu_{Si\text{–}O\text{–}Si}$ modes of the siliceous matrix of *MCM* and $\nu_{Si\text{–}O\text{–}Si}$ modes of the layers of the *K10* host clay are also present. In addition, for *K10nif*, bands corresponding to the $\nu_{Al\text{–}Al\text{–}OH}$, $\nu_{Al\text{–}O\text{–}Si}$ stretching modes, respectively, characteristic of the octahedral layer of the clay are also detected [61, 62].

Although the spectra of the composite materials *MCMnif* and *K10nif* are dominated by the bands of the host material, it is possible to see the presence of *Nif* owing to small, but relevant, spectral features that offer a positive identification of the guest. Still in Figure 4-top image shows spectral changes observed after drug loading. Therefore in *K10nif*, a set of three broad and very weak bands in the $\nu_{C\text{–}H}$ modes region (below 3000 cm^{-1}) indicate that *Nif* is present in the interlayer spacing of the host clay, without dramatic structural changes. The set of bands evidences that the drug was successfully loaded as well inside the pores of the *MCM* mesoporous material.

Comparison between the observed values found for *K10nif* and *MCMnif* shows that some bands are shifted. This situation may be due to the establishment of specific types of host-guest interactions (H-bond, ionic or other) between *Nif* and *K10* or *MCM* which will yield different release profiles, as discussed later in this chapter. In fact this is expected since *Nif* has carbonyl, amino and nitro groups which have electronegative oxygen and nitrogen centers (Figure 1). All these atoms hold electron lone pairs which can interact through hydrogen bonding with surface groups in *K10* or *MCM*.

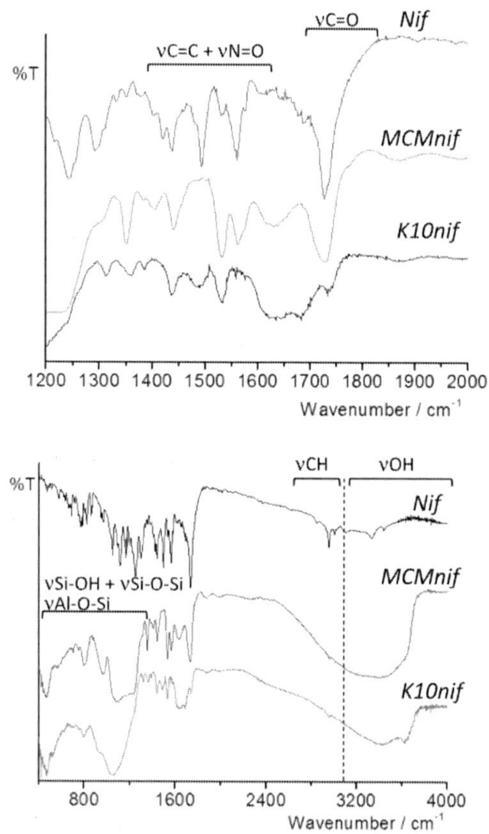

Figure 4. FTIR of pure *Nif* and composite materials *K10nif* and *MCMnif*: bottom – complete 400–4000 cm^{-1} range; top – zoom of the finger-print region.

This is probed especially in the case of *MCMnif* material by an intensity decrease of bands owing to Si–OH groups (Figure 4), upon drug loading indicating that the Si–OH surface groups of *MCM* are interacting with *Nif* molecules through those functional groups, as discussed recently by Xia *et al.* [63]. The sharp band arising from isolated OH groups has a much reduced intensity and the broad band assigned to H-bonded groups shows a red-shift (lower wavenumbers) and its profile is more complex [64] arising as well from hydrogen bonding with acceptor groups in *Nif* (carbonyl, amine and nitro). The carbonyl stretching region of *Nif* also shows evidence of intermolecular host-guest interaction, by displaying shifted bands in *K10nif* and *MCMnif* compared with neat *Nif* (Figure 4-top).

Further analysis of the FTIR of the composite materials reveals differences in the polymorphic form of *Nif* after immobilization inside the inorganic materials, compared to neat *Nif.* In this way, closer analysis of the finger print region (1200–1800 cm^{-1}) of neat *Nif* spectrum indicates that, according to the literature [65], the predominant form is α-*Nif*, being in excellent agreement with literature data [65]. In the case of *K10nif* and *MCMnif* there are differences not only between them but also with neat *Nif.* According to the corresponding vibrational spectra, differences may occur primarily from interactions arising from confinement effects leading to the establishment of hydrogen bonds among others. For *K10nif* composite material ionic interactions must be considered between the charged layers and the guest molecules. Comparing with the data described above for neat *Nif* it is clear that immobilization yields different molecular arrangements of the drug which are not compatible with the existence of α-*Nif.* Even the molecular arrangements between *K10nif* and *MCMnif* are shown to be different meaning that it is dependent on the matrix (either clay or the silica). Moreover the fingerprint regions of both *K10nif* and *MCMnif* composites show clear differences with broader bands in the former. This implies that interactions are stronger due to the charge balance effect (*Nif* behaves as a cation and *K10* has charge excess, described above). In both cases this may in fact be related to the different drug release profiles presented by these composite materials, with emphasis on the last period of drug release where the rate is driven by equilibrium between the carrier and functional groups of the drug molecules. This issue will be further addressed later in this chapter.

The XRD powder patterns of all host (*K10* and *MCM*) and composite (*K10nif* and *MCMnif*) materials are shown in Figure 5. For the clay system, most of the characteristic peaks in the two patterns are in the same position, except the characteristic peak indexed to the *001* reflection that is observed at $2\theta = 5.6°$ for *K10* and is shifted to $2\theta = 4.2°$ for *K10nif.*

According to Bragg's law, peaks shifting from higher to lower diffraction angles are explained by a *d*-spacing increase, which in this case changes from 15.8 Å to 21.0 Å after drug loading. Assuming that the alumino-silicate layer is ca. 9.6 Å thick [66], and according to simple molecular mechanics calculations, the maximum dimension of a *Nif* drug molecule is ca. 11 Å, including the solvent accessible radius (see Figure 1b). Therefore, from powder XRD data the gallery height is estimated to be 11.4 Å, and based on the largest dimension of *Nif* it is possible to estimate the tilt angle of the drug molecules in the interlayer gallery (α in Figure 6) as approximately 75°. This indicates that *Nif* molecules adopt an almost upright position. Taking this value into account, a proposal for the interlayer arrangement of the drug molecules is shown in Figure 6 (not at scale).

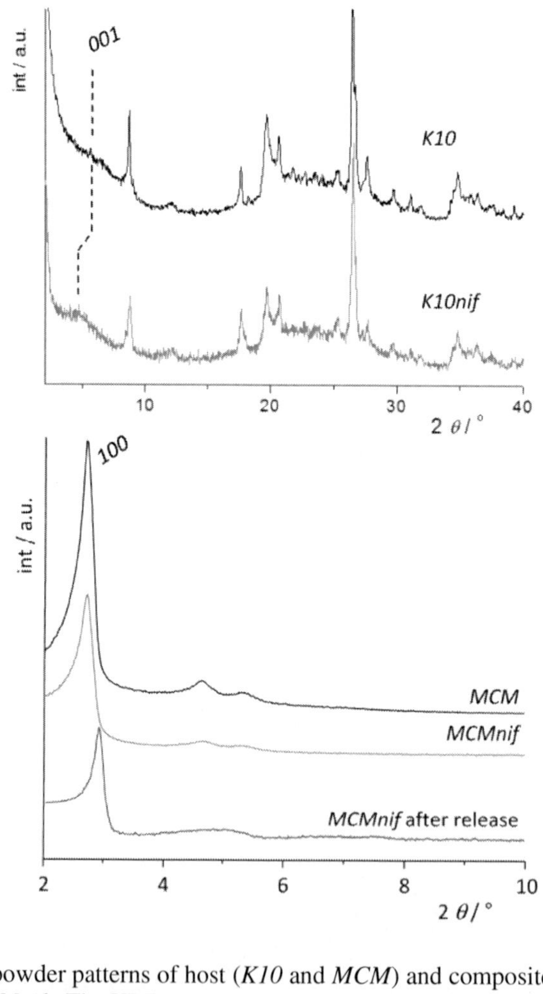

Figure 5. XRD powder patterns of host (*K10* and *MCM*) and composite materials (*K10nif* and *MCMnif*). The XRD powder pattern of the *MCMnif* material after drug release is also shown. The dashed line is an eye guide only.

As it results from a rough geometrical estimation, the proposed arrangement should be taken with care, since it depends on many other factors (humidity and temperature conditions) which were not accounted for.

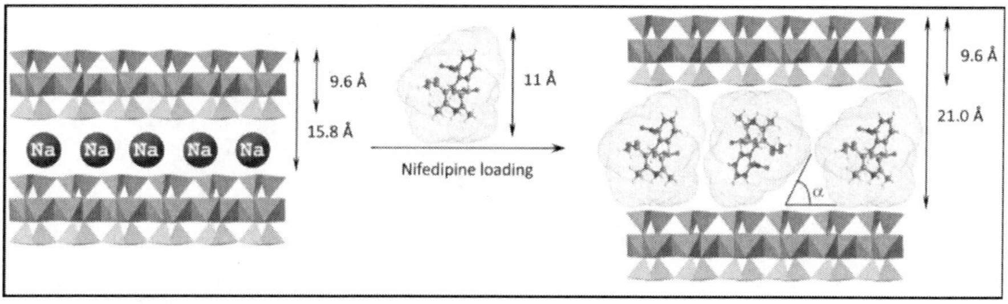

Figure 6. Schematic representation of *K10nif* composite material, showing a possible molecular arrangement of *Nif* inside the interlayer spacing. According to powder XRD data, α is the tilt angle of *Nif* being estimated to be 75°.

Considering now the *MCM* materials (Figure 5, bottom), the XRD powder pattern exhibits three reflections that are indexed to a hexagonal cell, the first corresponding to the *100* reflection, with *d* value of 32.2 Å. The XRD powder pattern of *MCMnif* is quite similar to that of *MCM*, which indicates retention of the long range hexagonal symmetry. There is a slight attenuation of XRD peak's intensities that must be interpreted most likely as being due to a reduction in the X-ray scattering contrast between the silica wall and the pore filling material (*Nif*) [67, 68].

The XRD powder patterns of *MCMnif* and *K10nif* after controlled drug release experiments are similar to those of the parent materials prior to intercalation. To this matter, it is known that mesoporous materials are not very stable under hydrothermal conditions, a process which is enhanced as temperature increases [69]. According to literature data, the mesoporous structure is not destroyed but rather suffers a process of dissolution/redeposition of $Si(OH)_4$ species. The result is probed as a decrease of both pore diameter and surface area, caused by the increased wall thickness arising from the above mentioned process. This is evidenced in Figure 5, by the XRD powder pattern which shows a shift towards higher 2θ values and also shows a decreased intensity.

Such findings are corroborated by results from electron microscopy – scanning electronic microscopy (SEM) and transmission electronic microscopy (TEM) – which will be discussed in the following lines of this chapter.

SEM and TEM imaging of the *MCMnif* and *K10nif* materials, before the release (Figures 7a, 7c, 7e and 7g) evidence the presence of a material with an ordered structure for *MCMnif* and a lamellar material for *K10nif*. In fact SEM images of both *MCMnif* and *K10nif* materials shows that particle morphology is somewhat similar, resembling irregular round shapes.

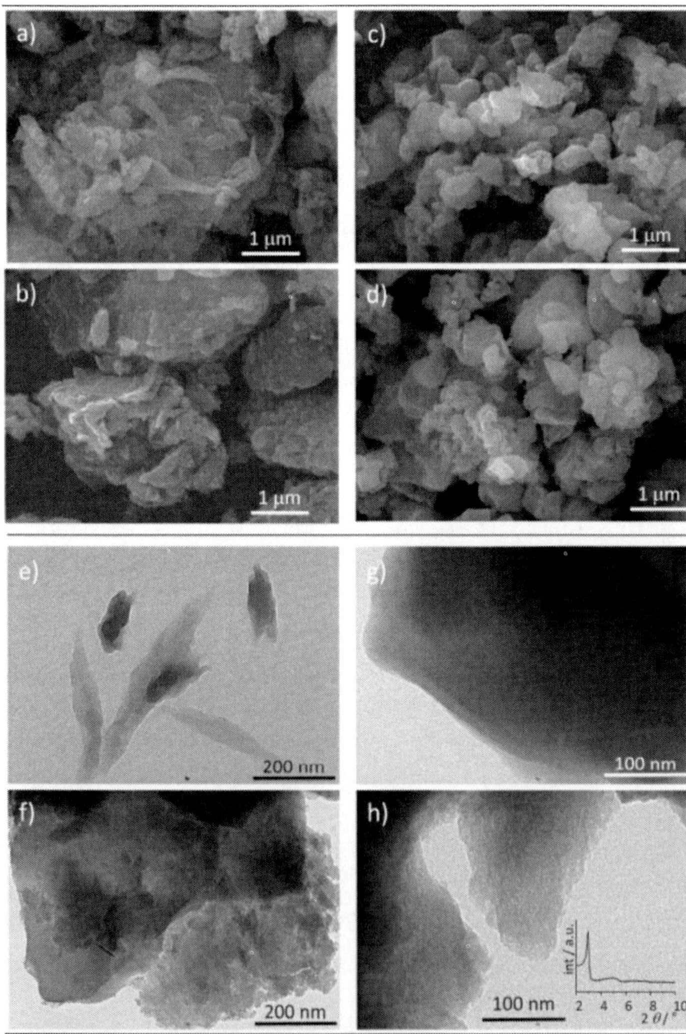

Figure 7. SEM [a) – d)] and TEM [e) – h)] images of *K10nif* [a) and e)] and *MCMnif* [c) and g)] before and of *K10nif* [b) and f)] and *MCMnif* [d) and h)] after drug release. The inset in Figure 7h shows the corresponding XRD powder pattern of the sample (same as on Figure 5).

After release experiments, SEM images of the resulting unloaded materials reveals that morphology has changed little. The main difference found is for the clay-based formulation – *K10nif* – which shows smaller particles coating the original host material larger grains. EDS analysis to this material after drug release revealed the presence of calcium, which may indicate initial formation of hydroxyapatite on the surface of *K10* (the presence of phosphorous could not be confirmed since the loading might be below the detection limit). This situation arises from the fact that the SBF where the release experiment is conducted has calcium in its formulation. This is surely a very important feature of this material showing that it can be biocompatible. On the contrary, EDS analysis on *MCMnif* did not reveal the presence of any amount of calcium. TEM imaging of *K10nif* before and after drug release experiments did evidence quite some changes. In fact while *K10nif* is composed mainly of small needle-like crystalline particles, after drug release the particles although retaining its needle-like form, are now coated with a large mass that glues them across large areas. This may be due to the formation of the above mentioned structures containing calcium, as detected by EDS analysis.

In the case of *MCMnif*, TEM images show that the array of ordered channels is detected in this material being maintained as well after drug has been released. As can be seen in Figure 7, before and after drug release, mesoporous channels are easily observed, confirming that, to some extent, this material is resistant to the conditions used. However, this does not make proof of the channel structure preservation to its initial stage. As discussed above, the XRD powder pattern of *MCM* after drug release shows that although its primary structure is preserved it has suffered hydrothermal degradation. Figure7h includes the XRD powder pattern of the material after release.

Figure 8 shows the thermogravimetric analyses (TGA) of all materials (host and composite) discussed in the present work and including the thermal profile of *Nif* as well. Both *MCM* and *K10* host materials show mass losses till 200 °C corresponding to physisorbed water. After this temperature only a negligible mass amount is still lost by both *MCM* and *K10* materials, most probably due to dehydroxylation. TGA analysis of *Nif* shows a two-step degradation process, the first one occurring between 120–500 °C and the second between 500–800 °C with a total mass loss of ca. 88%.

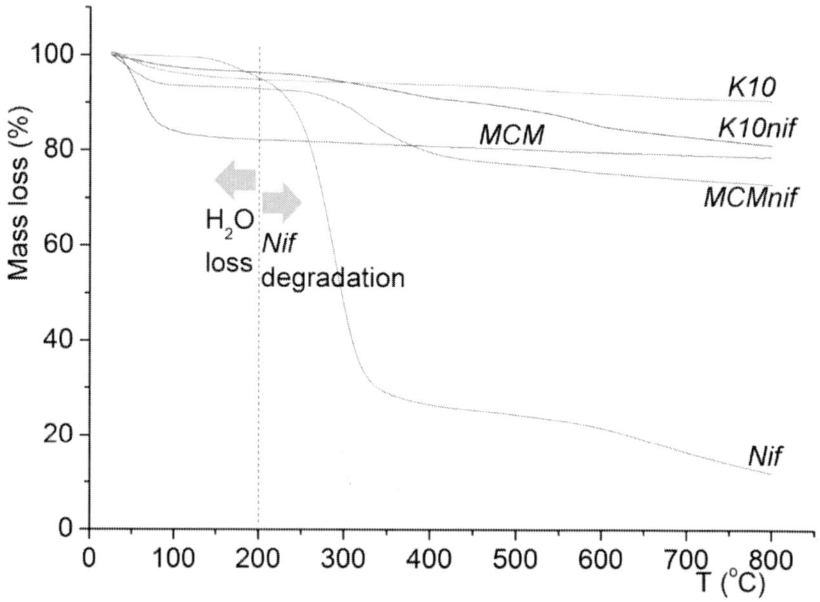

Figure 8. TGA profiles for *Nif*, *K10*, *K10nif*, *MCM*, and *MCMnif* materials. The dashed line is an eye-guide to distinguish major zones concerning H_2O desorption and *Nif* degradation.

In what concerns the *K10nif* and *MCMnif* composite materials the loss of physisorbed water is also observed till 200 °C, reaching a content of 5-7%. Afterwards the same two-step mass loss, in the 200–800 °C range is observed, corresponding to the gradual decomposition of *Nif*. Considering also the fact that mass losses start at higher temperatures than observed for neat *Nif* (200 °C vs. 120 °C), this can be interpreted as a suggestion that the drug is mostly inside either the intragallery spacing of *K10* or the mesopores of *MCM* materials. This result evidences as well that both *K10nif* and *MCMnif* composite materials are good thermic stabilizers of the drug which make the formulation to resist better against environmental conditions (either heat or moisture). This is in agreement with published data concerning vitrification of *Nif* inside a xerogel where the same behavior is observed [35].

According to Figure 1b the approximate area of *Nif* molecule amounts to c.a. 1.05 nm^2. For covering an *MCM* mesopore average surface area of *ca.* 900 $m^2\ g^{-1}$ with a monolayer of *Nif*, a theoretical loading of c.a. 49.3 % is required. However, the observed loading corresponds to 19.7 % loading with a water content of 7 %, which corresponds to only *ca.* 40 % of the saturation loading, in line with literature data [64, 70, 71]. This value agrees with the fact that *Nif* is adsorbed inside *MCM* in a different crystalline form than in neat form, thus corroborating with FTIR data, as discussed earlier in this chapter. This also evidences that *MCM* is an adequate support to poor soluble drugs, in line with other reports found in the literature [64, 70, 71].

A final word should be given to the beneficial effects of hosting *Nif* drug inside the host materials herein described. This is of major importance when developing formulations where one cannot only think of the delivery performance (which is a mandatory objective) but one has to care also about drug stability. In this way to evaluate the advantageous effect of the formulated materials *K10nif* and *MCMnif*, simple experiments have also been carried out. Samples of each of both materials were split into two sets. One was exposed for a month to indirect sunlight (denoted *exposed*) and the other set was kept for 18 months in a closed vessel under regular atmosphere and in the dark. Afterwards, the drug was extracted and analyzed by GC-MS and compared with neat *Nif* drug as control. The result, shown in Figure 9, evidenced by the chromatograms of the samples stored either in the dark for 18 months or exposed for a month to indirect sunlight match perfectly the chromatogram of the control sample. This is indeed an advantageous property of the immobilization of *Nif* inside *K10* and *MCM*.

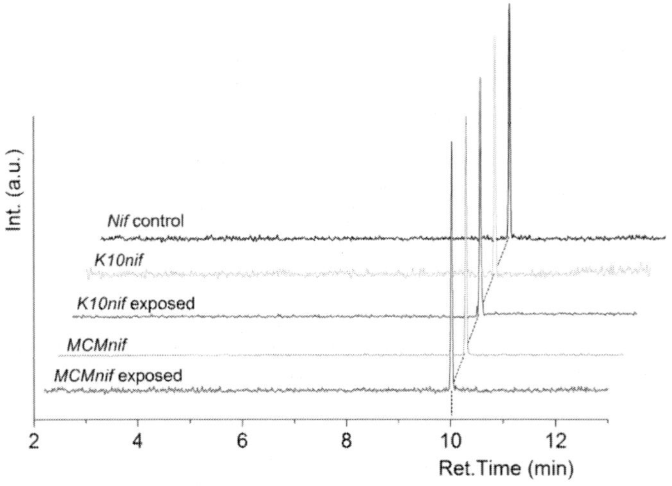

Figure 9. GC chromatograms of *Nif* drug released from *K10nif* and *MCMnif* materials after being kept under different conditions: *K10nif* and *MCMnif* lines refer to samples stored for 18 months under regular atmosphere in a closed vessel and in the dark; *K10nif* exposed and *MCMnif* exposed lines were stored under indirect sunlight for one month. Also shown is the chromatogram for *Nif* neat drug as control, showing that all are comparable. Dashed line is eye-guide only.

Drug Release Profiles

The *in vitro* drug release profiling was assessed by conducting experiments using a simulated body fluid (SBF) to simulate *in vivo* circulation fluid. Drug release profiling was carried out by incubating composite materials during 20 h at 37 °C [72].

Typical drug release profiles for the different types of investigated materials, *K10nif* and *MCMnif*, are plotted in Figure 10. The controlled release tests were carried out suspending the composite materials under continuous stirring at the temperature of 37±0.1 °C in a simulated body fluid (SBF), at pH 7.4, maintaining an initial ratio of ml_{SBF}/mg_{Nif} absorbed set to 1. Since this ratio was initially set to 1, the 100% mark in Figure 10 corresponds to the complete release of *Nif* drug from the carriers. This means that in a complete release test a concentration of 1 mg_{Nif}/ml_{SBF} in solution would be measured. In order to keep this ratio, and according with *Nif* loading data (see earlier discussion in this chapter) the amount of *K10nif* reaches *ca.* 7.2 mg_{Nif}/ml_{SBF} and for *MCMnif* there is the need to use *ca.* 4.1 mg_{Nif}/ml_{SBF}.

The results represented in Figure 10 show that after a period of 20 h none of the samples (*MCMnif* and *K10nif*) has completely released the drug, similarly to results reported recently for delivery of other drugs (gentamicin) [63].

This fact is less significant in the release profile of *MCMnif*, where the release ratio reaches ca. 50% after 20 h. On the other hand, controlled release from *K10nif* composite is even poorer leading only to a small amount of the initial *Nif* loading as low as 31%.

In the *K10nif* composite, the low release amount may be explained by the existence of stronger interactions between the protonated amino group of *Nif* and the anionic groups from the layers of *K10* clay [54, 73]. This is corroborated by FTIR data (see Figure 4), where bands due to the guest drug clearly show broad profiles, probing intermolecular interactions and probably stronger than found in *MCMnif*, which shows narrower band profiles. For the latter, *MCMnif*, interactions between host-guest species can be assumed to be established mainly by means of hydrogen bonding between the guest molecule and the silanol groups at the surface of the host material. Therefore, the weaker host-guest interactions should contribute to a more extensive release of the guest in this case, which is in fact observed. A similar situation has already been described previously by Vallet-Regi and co-workers, while studying MCM-41 loaded with ibuprofen [74]. Still on this topic, very recently Ukmar *et al.* reported the study of interactions occurring inside pore walls in mesoporous materials. In that work it was reported that specific host wall-guest drug interactions (i.e. hydrogen bonds) may affect the effective transfer of drug into bulk solution [75]. By the same token in the case of clays (*K10nif*), the interactions are also responsible for the different kinetics, as discussed above.

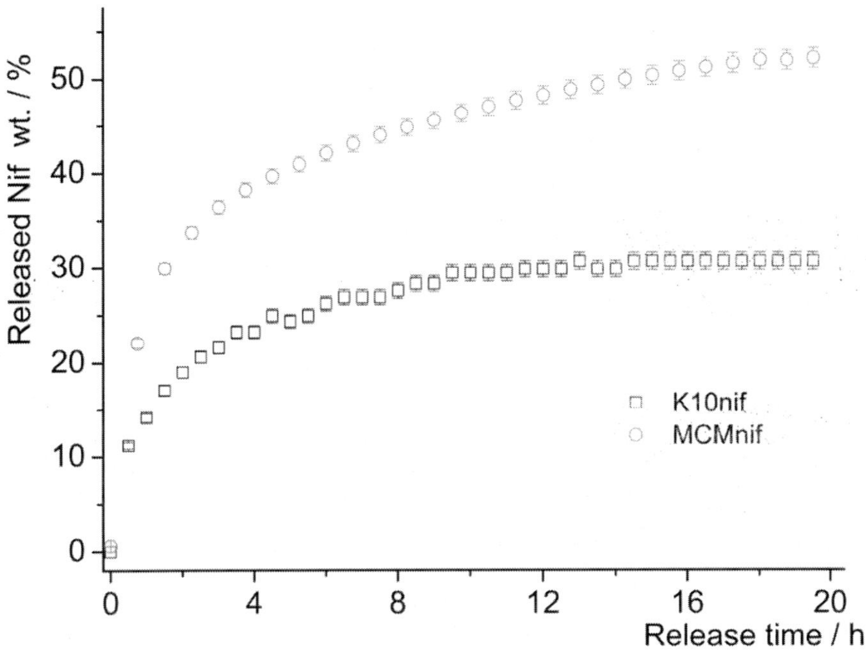

Figure 10. Drug release profiles (error bars are included) of both composite materials at 37 °C in a simulated body fluid (SBF).

Yet another critical factor that should be taken into account is drug solubility in the medium. Although *Nif* is known to exhibit low and concomitantly pH dependent solubility, the fact that the release is done slowly and that the SBF itself contains different ions, it is expected that this issue may be minimized. In addition, the specific interactions discussed above may also be regarded as a beneficial effect (to some extent), since a somewhat delayed release may account for a smoother solubility minimizing insolubility issues due to local high concentration areas.

The release rate of *Nif* from the host matrices was found to be higher for *MCMnif* than for *K10nif*. Specifically, the initial delivery rates (calculated in the first 2 h of release) were calculated to be 0.42 $mg{\cdot}h^{-1}$ for *K10nif* and 0.57

$mg{\cdot}h^{-1}$ for *MCMnif* relatively to *Nif*. These values are equivalent to the complete release of 3.0 $mg{\cdot}h^{-1}$ and 2.40 $mg{\cdot}h^{-1}$ for *MCMnif* as formulated for *K10nif* and for *MCMnif*, respectively. Initial release rates were determined by fitting the absorbance vs. time data to Eq. (1):

$$N_t = N_\infty (1 - e^{k \cdot t}) \quad (1)$$

where N_t and N_∞ are the quantities of *Nif* at time t and at the end of release, respectively, k representing the calculated release rate.

MCMnif shows a higher initial capacity of delivering the loading to the biological medium at any given time interval compared to *K10nif*. This shows, together with the maximum amount of drug delivered, that the *MCM* matrix is more effective for both rapid drug delivery in a short term period and for a prolonged treatment, where after the 20 h period a well-defined plateau has not been reached. This may indicate that continuous release may be achieved as the released drug is being consumed from the medium. On the contrary, the release profile of *K10nif* leads to a plateau ca. 8 h after administration. From these observations it is assumed that *MCMnif* can be an effective alternative for a one day administration as it can release the drug almost constantly during such period.

In parallel, similar controlled release experiments were carried out in Petri dishes using the same conditions, but under static conditions (no stirring). This makes the release process mainly diffusion-controlled, but allows a visual perception of the release performance for both composite materials, benchmarked by neat *Nif*. Drug release was visually controlled by adding some drops of a KOH solution to the incubated dishes which will yield a yellow color if *Nif* is present [76]. All images were taken after 24 h incubation time. It is obvious for the case of *K10nif* (Figure 11, top image) that release is deficient (almost colorless solution) compared with that observed for *MCMnif* and neat *Nif*, both of them showing a strong yellow color from released *Nif* to SBF medium. Such observations confirm the kinetic data described above.

Another relevant feature that was observed is the fact that when using *MCMnif* composite (Figure 11, middle image) as the drug carrier, the apparent solubility (or released amount of *Nif*) is found to be higher than that observed when using neat *Nif* (Figure 11, bottom image). This fact may possibly arise from two phenomena either isolated or combined. The first is that the measured release rate of *Nif* from *MCMnif* may be slow enough (although faster than *K10nif*) to allow extra solubility of the drug in the SBF medium.

The other one is that when *Nif* is loaded inside *MCM* pores it may be crystallized in a form that shows higher solubility, such as amorphous, which is known to have higher solubility [77] and has been described to be the only possible polymorph that can be crystallized inside pores of such dimensions [35].

It should also be mentioned that for *K10nif* to reach some amount of detectable *Nif* (Figure 11, inset in the top image) through this method, the release experiment took as much as 108 h, stressing the low efficiency of this composite in performing such task.

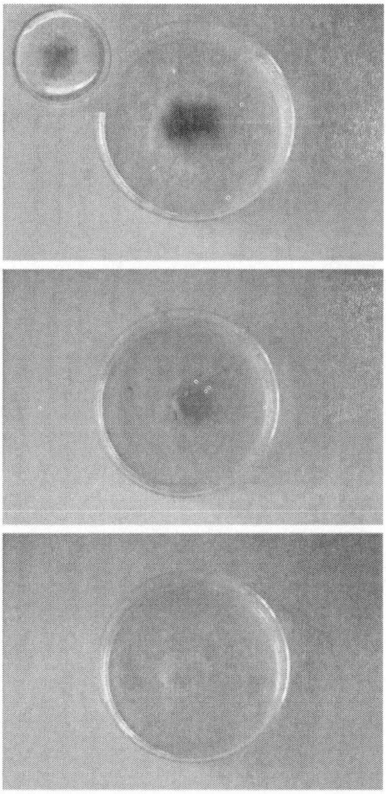

Figure 11. Photographs of the SBF medium for testing the efficiency of *K10nif* (top), *MCMnif* (middle) as drug delivery systems, during a 20 h release experiment. Control experiment was carried out repeating the same experiment with neat *Nif* (bottom). The inset in the top image refers to the same experiments using *K10nif*, but after 108 h release time. All experiments were carried out at 37 °C. Nif release to the SBF medium was probed adding a few drops of 2M KOH, yielding a yellow color when and where *Nif* is present.

Taking the best performing drug delivery system discussed here, *MCMnif*, and comparing it with a recently reported system based on nanofibers [78], the latter was reported to be able to release almost 100% of the loaded drug. Although it was found to be pH dependent as evidenced by tests simulating gastrointestinal pH environments. Nonetheless, results described here refer to the behavior of the drug delivery system in SBF, simulating the circulatory system to evaluate how it will behave under such conditions. Despite this, and concerning only the released drug amount, it should be mentioned that the previously reported nanofiber drug delivery system is based on a micro-scale pore system whereas that of *MCM* is based on a nano-scale one, which certainly is relevant to the differences observed.

Conclusion

The present chapter aimed at an overview of recent literature concerning the use of inorganic materials as matrices for nifedipine (*Nif*) and their use as drug delivery systems. The current state of the art shows that there are not many devoted studies on this drug, but potential is high.

To give the reader the power to evaluate such systems, a case study comparing two different matrices was presented and discussed. *Nif*, a calcium channel blocker, was loaded in *K10*, a microporous clay, and *MCM*, a mesoporous material with a hexagonal array of the channels.

Careful characterization of the materials made possible to assess the existence of different kinds of intermolecular host-guest interactions, depending on the host used – *K10* or *MCM*. This is relevant at the stage of testing the drug delivery systems, which yield different release kinetics for both materials. In addition, electron microscopy imaging shows that both host materials are adequate to perform this function as little changes are observed. EDS analysis show that *K10* after release experiments has calcium in its composition which may arise from the formation of hydroxyapatite, rendering such material important biocompatibility properties.

The composite materials behave differently concerning drug release. *MCMnif* has faster release kinetics, and delivers higher quantities of *Nif* compared to *K10nif* composite. In fact, after 20 h, the kinetic profile of *MCMnif* still does not show a plateau, which indicates that drug delivery is performed continuously throughout the whole experiment time and leading to an ideal administration of a single daily dose. In addition it was confirmed that the *MCM* is capable of achieving higher drug loadings (ca. 50% higher mol loading) and concomitantly releasing it in higher availability than found for the *K10* clay.

In addition, drug solubility seems also to be a relevant issue as the results from *MCMnif* show that the delivered amount into the SBF medium is higher than that found using neat *Nif* as control. This is also an advantageous feature that could help to resolve an important issue in drug bioavailability.

Furthermore, it was also found that the hybrid formulation materials work also as a stabilizing agent for drug storing. The composite materials show enhanced photostabilization of the drug after immobilization inside the host materials. This was confirmed by GC/MS analyses on samples stored for at least eighteen months, which denotes a major improvement over neat *Nif*, which is known to undergo easy photodegradation.

References

[1] Muller, JE; Gunther SJ. Nifedipine therapy for Prinzmetal's angina, *Circulation*, 1978, 57, 137-139.

[2] Bertrand, ME; Lablanche, JM; Tilmant, PY. Treatment of prinzmetal's variant angina: Role of medical treatment with nifedipine and surgical coronary revascularization combined with plexectomy, *American Journal of Cardiology*, 1981, 47, 174–178.

[3] Hasegawa, A; Nakagawa, H; Sugimoto, I. Bioavailability and stability of nifedipine-enteric coating agent solid dispersion, *Chemical Pharmaceutical Bulletin*,1985, 33, 388–391.

[4] Hasegawa, A; Kawamura, R; Nakagawa, H; Sugimoto, I. Physical properties of solid dispersions of poorly water-soluble drugs with enteric coating agents, *Chemical Pharmaceutical Bulletin*, 1985, 33, 3429–3435.

[5] Hasegawa, A; Nakagawa, H; Sugimoto, I. Application of solid dispersions of nifedipine with enteric coating agent to prepare a sustained-release dosage form, *Chemical Pharmaceutical Bulletin*, 1985, 33, 1615-1619.

[6] Mitchell, SA; Reynolds, TD; Dasbach, TP. A compaction process to enhance dissolution of poorly water-soluble drugs using hydroxypropyl methylcellulose, *International Journal of Pharmaceutics*, 2003, 250, 3–11.

[7] Sugimoto, I; Sasaki, K; Kuchiki, A; Ishihara, T; Nakagawa, H. Stability and bioavailability of nifedipine in fine granules, *Chemical Pharmaceutical Bulletin*, 1982,30, 4479–4488.

[8] Zajc, N; Obreza, A; Bele, M; Srcic, S. Physical properties and dissolution behaviour of nifedipine/mannitol solid dispersions prepared by hot melt method, *International Journal of Pharmaceutics*, 2005, 291, 51–58.

[9] Chutimaworapan, S; Ritthidej, GC; Yonemochi, E; Oguchi, T; Yamamoto, K. Effect of water-soluble carriers on dissolution characteristics of nifedipine solid dispersions, *Drug Development and Industrial Pharmacy*, 2000, 26, 1141–1150.

[10] Bayomi, MA; Abanumay, KA; Al-Angary, AA. Effect of inclusion complexation with cyclodextrins on photostability of nifedipine in solid state, *International Journal of Pharmaceutics*, 2002, 243,107– 117.

[11] Hecq, J; Deleers, M; Fanara, D; Vranckx, H; Amighi, K. Preparation and characterization of nanocrystals for solubility and dissolution rate enhancement of nifedipine, *International Journal of Pharmaceutics*, 2005, 299, 167–177.

[12] Kerc, J; Srcic, S; Knez, Z; Sencar-Bozic, P. Micronization of drugs using supercritical carbon dioxide, *International Journal of Pharmaceutics*, 1999, 182, 33–39.

[13] Gupta, H; Bhandari, D; Sharma, A. Recent trends in oral drug delivery: a review, *Recent Patents on Drug Delivery & Formulation*, 2009, 3, 162-173.

[14] Sastry, SV; Nyshadham, JR; Fix, JA. Recent technological advances in oral drug delivery – a review, *Pharmaceutical Science & Technology Today*, 2000, 3, 138–145.

[15] Colombo, P; Sonvico, F; Colombo, G; Bettini, R. Novel platforms for oral drug delivery, *Pharmaceutical Research*, 2009, 26, 601–611.

[16] *Encyclopedic Handbook of Biomaterials and Bioengineering*. New York: Marcel Dekker, Inc; 1995.

[17] Hyakuna, K; Yamamuro, T; Kotoura, Y; Oka, M; Nakamura, T; Kitsugi, T; Kokubo, T; Kushitani, H. Surface reactions of calcium phosphate ceramics to various solutions, *Journal of Biomedical Materials Research Part A*, 1990, 24, 471– 488.

[18] Suzuki, T; Arai, K; Goto, H; Hanano, M; Watanabe, J; Tomono, K. Dissolution tests for self-setting calcium phosphate cement-containing nifedipine, *Chemical Pharmaceutical Bulletin*, 2002, 50, 741-743.

[19] Yanagisawa, T; Shimizu, T; Kuroda, K; Kato, C. The preparation of alkyltrimethylammnonium–kanemite complexes and their conversion to microporous materials, *Bulletin of the Chemical Society of Japan*, 1990, 63, 988-992.

[20] Inagaki, S; Fukushima, Y; Kuroda, K. Synthesis of highly ordered mesoporous materials from a layered polysilicate, *Journal of the Chemical Society – Chemical Communications*, 1993, 8, 680-681.

[21] Kresge, CT; Leonowicz, ME; Roth, WJ; Vartuli, JC; Beck, JS. Ordered mesoporous molecular sieves synthesized by a liquid-crystal template mechanism, *Nature*, 1992, 359, 710-712.

[22] Hoffmann, F; Cornelius, M; Morell, J; Fröba, M. Silica-based mesoporous organic–inorganic hybrid materials, *Angewandte Chemie International Edition*, 2006, 45, 3216-3251.

[23] Ford, DM; Simanek, EE; Shantz, DF. Engineering nanospaces: ordered mesoporous silicas as model substrates for building complex hybrid materials, *Nanotechnology,* 2005, 16, S458-S475.

[24] Vallet-Regi, M; Balas, F; Arcos, D. Mesoporous materials for drug delivery, *Angewandte Chemie International Edition*, 2007, 46, 7548-7558.

[25] Manzano, M; Colilla, M; Vallet-Regi, M. Drug delivery from ordered mesoporous matrices, *Expert Opinion on Drug Delivery*, 2009, 6, 1383-1400.

[26] Dua, P; Chaudhari, KN; Lee, CH; Chaudhari, NK; Hong, SW; Yu, JS; Kim, S; Lee, DK. Evaluation of toxicity and gene expression changes triggered by oxide nanoparticles, *Bulletin of the Korean Chemical Society*, 2011, 32, 2051-2057.

[27] Kortesuo, P; Ahola, M; Karlsson, S; Kangasniemi, I; Yli-Urpo, A; Kiesvaara, J. Silica xerogel as an implantable carrier for controlled drug delivery – evaluation of drug distribution and tissue effects after implantation, *Biomaterials*, 2000, 21, 193-198.

[28] Ahola, M; Kortesuo, P; Kangasniemi, I; Kiesvaara, J; Yli-Urpo, A. Silica xerogel carrier material for controlled release of toremifene citrate, *International Journal of Pharmaceutics*, 2000, 195, 219-227.

[29] Nicoll, SB; Radin, S. In vitro release kinetics of biologically active transforming growth factor-1 from novel porous glass carrier, *Biomaterials*, 18, 853-859.

[30] Santos, EM; Radin, S. Sol-gel delivered carrier for controlled release of proteins, *Biomaterials*, 20, 1695-1700.

[31] Böttcher, H; Slowik, P; Süß, W. Sol-gel carrier systems for controlled drug delivery, *Journal of Sol-Gel Science and Technology*, 1998, 13, 277-281.

[32] Morais, EC; Correa, GG; Brambilla, R; Radtke, C; Baibich, IM; Santos, JHZ. The interaction of encapsulated pharmaceutical drugs with a silica matrix, *Colloids and Surfaces B: Biointerfaces*, 2013, 103, 422-429.

[33] Maver, U; Godec, A; Bele, M; Planinšek, O; Gaberšček, S; Jamnik, J. Novel hybrid silica xerogels for stabilization and controlled release of drug, *International Journal of Pharmaceutics*, 2007, 330, 164-174.

[34] Tran, PH-L; Tran, TT-D; Lee, K-H, Kim, D-J; Lee, B-J. Dissolution-modulating mechanism of pH modifiers in solid dispersion containing weakly acidic or basic drugs with poor water solubility, *Expert Opinion on Drug Delivery*, 2010, 10, 647-661.

[35] Godec, A; Maver, U; Bele, M; Planinšek, O; Srčič, S; Gaberšček, M; Jamnik, J. Vitrification from solution in restricted space: Formation and stabilization of amorphous nifedipine in a nanoporous silica xerogel carrier, *International Journal of Pharmaceutics*, 2007, 343, 131-140.

[36] Speibroeck, MV; Barillaro, V; Thi, TD; Mellaerts, R; Martens, J; Humbeeck, JV; Vermant, J; Annaert, P; Mooter, GVD; Augustinjs, P. Ordered mesoporous silica material sba-15: a broad-spectrum formulation platform for poorly soluble drugs, *Journal of Phamaceutical Sciences*, 2009, 98, 2648-2658.

[37] Friedrich, H; Fussnegger, B; Kolter, K; Bodmeier, R. Dissolution rate improvement of poorly water-soluble drugs obtained by adsorbing solutions of drugs, in hydrophilic solvents onto high surface are carriers, *European Journal of Pharmaceutics & Biopharmaceutics* 2006, 62, 171-177.

[38] Fernandes, CI; Nunes, CD; Vaz, PD. Clays in organic synthesis–preparation and catalytic applications, *Current Organic Synthesis*, 2012, 9, 670-694.

[39] Lerf, A. Different modes and consequences of electron transfer in intercalation compounds. *Journal of Physics and Chemistry of Solids*, 2004, 65, 553-563.

[40] Bruce, DW; O´Hare, D. In: *Inorganic Materials*, John Wiley and Sons Ed.; England, 1992, pp.166-235.

[41] Kryszewski, M. Nanointercalates-novel class of materials with promising properties. *Synthetic Metals,* 2000, 109, 47-54.

[42] Alexandre, M; Dubois, P. Polymer-layered silicate nanocomposites: preparation, properties and uses of a new class of materials. *Materials Science & Eng*ineering, 2000, 28, 1-63.

[43] Brindley, GW; Brown, G. *Crystal Structure of Clay Materials and their X-ray identification*; Mineralogical Society: London, 1980.

[44] Ramesh, TN; Rajamathi, M; Kamath, PV. Ammonia induced precipitation of cobalt hydroxide: observation of turbostratic disorder. *Solid State Sciences,* 2003, 5, 751-756.

[45] Klein, C; Hurlbut, CS. I*n: Manual of Mineralogy,* John Wiley & Sons Ed.; England, 1993, pp. 392-398.

[46] *Layered Double Hydroxides: Present and Future*, Nova Science Publishers Ed.; New York, 2001.

[47] Carlino, S. The intercalation of carboxylic acids into layered double hydroxides: a critical evaluation and review of the different methods, *Solid State Ionics*, 1997*, 98*, 73-84.

[48] Crepaldi, L.; Valim, J.B. Hidróxidos duplos lamelares: síntese, estrutura, propriedades e aplicações. *Química Nova*, 1998, 21, 300-311.

[49] Lagaly, G. Introduction: From clay mineral-polymer interactions to clay mineral-polymer nanocomposites, *Applied Clay Science,* 1999, 15, 1-9.

[50] Matsumura, A; Komori, Y; Itagaki, T; Sugahara, Y; Kuroda, K. Preparation of a kaolinite–nylon 6 intercalation compound, *Bulletin of the Chemical Society of Japan*, 2001, 74, 1153−1158.

[51] Pomogailo, AD. Hybrid intercalative nanocomposites, *Inorganic Materials*, 2005*, 41,* S47-S74.

[52] Rajamathi, M; Thomas, GS; Kamath, PV. The many ways of making anionic clays, *Proceedings of the Indian Academy of Sciences (Chemical Sciences)*, 2001, 113, 671–680.

[53] Park, KW; Kwon, OY. Interlamellar silylation of montmorillonite with 3-aminopropyltriethoxysilane, *Bulletin of the Korean Chemical Society*, 2004, 25, 965-968.

[54] Lin, FH; Lee, YH; Jian, CH; Wong, JM; Shieh, MJ; Wang, CY. A study of purified montmorillonite intercalated with 5-fluorouracil as drug carrier, *Biomaterials*, 2002, 23, 1981-1987.

[55] Lee, YH; Kuo, TF; Chen, BY; Feng, YK; Wen, YR; Lin, WC; Lin, FH. Toxicity assessment of montmorillonite as a drug carrier for pharmaceutical applications: yeast and rats model, *Biomedical Engineering: Applications, Basis and Communications*, 2005, 17, 72-78.

[56] EFSA Panel on Additives and Products or Substances used in animal feed (FEEDAP), *EFSA Journal*, 2011, 9, 2007-2030.

[57] Vaz, PD; Nunes, CD. A new role for layered double hydroxides hybrid materials—uptake and delivery of small molecules into the gas phase, *New Journal of Chemistry*, 2010, 34, 541-546.

[58] Palmer, SJ; Frost, RL; Nguyen, T. Hydrotalcites and their role in coordination of anions in Bayer liquors: Anion binding in layered double hydroxides, *Coordination Chemistry Reviews,* 2009, 253, 250-267.

[59] Debecker, DP; Gaigneaux, EM; Busca, G. Exploring, tuning, and exploiting the basicity of hydrotalcites for applications in heterogeneous catalysis. *Chemistry – A European Journal,* 2009, 15, 3920-3935.

[60] Veerabadran, NG; Price, RR; Lvov, YM. Clay nanotubes for encapsulation and sustained release of drugs, *NANO: Brief Reports and Reviews*, 2007, 2, 115-120.

[61] Komadel, P; Bujdak, J; Madejova, J; Sucha, V; Elsass, F. Effect of non-swelling layers on the dissolution of reduced-charge montmorillonite in hydrochloric acid, *Clay Minerals*, 1996, 31, 333-345.

[62] Nasser, A; Gal, M; Gerstl, Z; Mingelgrin, U; Yariv, S. Adsorption of alachlor by montmorillonites, *Journal of Thermal Analysis and Calorimetry*, 1997, 50, 257-268.

[63] Xia, W; Chang, J. Well-ordered mesoporous bioactive glasses (MBG): A promising bioactive drug delivery system, *Journal of Controlled Release,* 2006, 110, 522-530.

[64] Mellaerts, R; Roeffaers, MBJ; Houthoofd, K; Van Speybroeck, M; De Cremer, G; Jammaer, JAG; Van den Mooter, G; Augustijns, P; Hofkens, J; Martens, JA. Molecular organization of hydrophobic molecules and co-adsorbed water in SBA-15 ordered mesoporous silica material, *Physical Chemistry Chemical Physics*, 2011, 13, 2706-2713.

[65] Chan, KLA; Fleming, OS; Kazarian, SG; Vassou, D; Chryssikos, GD; Gionis, V, Polymorphism and devitrification of nifedipine under controlled humidity: a combined FT-Raman, IR and Raman microscopic investigation, *Journal of Raman Spectroscopy*, 2004, 35, 353-359.

[66] Ohtsuka, K. Preparation and properties of two-dimensional microporous pillared interlayered solids, *Chemistry of Materials*, 1997, 9, 2039-2050.

[67] Marler, B; Oberhagemann, U; Vortmann, S; Gies, H. Influence of the sorbate type on the XRD peak intensities of loaded MCM-41, *Microporous Materials*, 1996, 6, 375-383.

[68] Hammond, W; Prouzet, E; Mahanti, SD; Pinnavaia, TJ. Structure factor for the periodic walls of mesoporous MCM-41 molecular sieves, *Microporous Mesoporous Materials*, 1999, 27, 19-25.

[69] Galarneau, A; Nader, M; Guenneau, F; Di Renzo, F; Gedeon, A. Understanding the stability in water of mesoporous SBA-15 and MCM-41, *Journal of Physical Chemistry C*, 2007, 111, 8268-8277.

[70] Mellaerts,R; Aerts, CA; Van Humbeeck, J; Augustijns, P; Van den Mooter, G; Martens, J.A. Enhanced release of itraconazole from ordered mesoporous SBA-15 silica materials, *Chemical Communications*, 2007, 1375-1377.

[71] Mellaerts, R; Houthoofd, K; Elen, K; Chen, H; Van Speybroeck, M; Van Humbeeck, J; Augustijns, P; Mullens, J; Van den Mooter, G; Martens, JA. Aging behavior of pharmaceutical formulations of itraconazole on SBA-15 ordered mesoporous silica carrier material, *Microporous and Mesoporous Materials* 2010, 130, 154-161.

[72] Nunes, CD; Vaz, PD; Fernandes, AC; Ferreira, P; Romão, CC; Calhorda, MJ. Loading and delivery of sertraline using inorganic micro and mesoporous materials, *European Journal of Pharmaceutics and Biopharmaceutics*, 2007, 66, 357-365.

[73] Kollar, T; Palinko, I; Konya, Z; Kiricsi, I. Intercalating amino acid guests into montmorillonite host, *Journal of Molecular Structure*, 2003, 651, 335-340.

[74] Muñoz, B; Ramila, A; Perez-Pariente, J; Diaz, I; Vallet-Regi, M. MCM-41 organic modification as drug delivery rate regulator, *Chemistry of Materials*, 2003, 15, 500-503.

[75] Ukmar, T; Maver, U; Planinšek, O; Kaučič, V; Gaberšček, M; Godec, A. Understanding controlled drug release from mesoporous silicates: Theory and experiment, *Journal of Controlled Release*, 2011, 155, 409-417.

[76] Rahman, N; Azmi, SNH. New spectrophotometric methods for the determination of nifedipine in pharmaceutical formulations, *Acta Biochimica Polonica*, 2005, 52, 915-922.

[77] Lalitha, Y; Lakshmi, PK. Enhancement of dissolution of nifedipine by surface solid dispersion technique, *International Journal of Pharmacy and Pharmaceutical Sciences*, 2011, 3, 41-46.

[78]] Park, CG; Kim, E; Park, M; Park, J-H; Choy, YB. A nanofibrous sheet-based system for linear delivery of nifedipine, *Journal of Controlled Release*, 2011, 149, 250-257.

Index

D

G

H

I

J

K

L

M

N

O

P

Q

R

S

T

U

V

W

X

Y

Z